Neighborhood Psychiatry

Neighborhood Psychiatry

Edited by

Lee B. Macht, M.D.
The Harvard Medical School

Donald J. Scherl, M.D.
The Harvard Medical School

Steven Sharfstein, M.D.
National Institute of Mental Health

Lexington Books

D.C. Heath and Company
Lexington, Massachusetts
Toronto

Library of Congress Cataloging in Publication Data

Main entry under title:

Neighborhood psychiatry.

   Includes index.
   1. Community mental health. 2. Social psychiatry. I. Macht,
Lee B. II. Scherl, Donald J. III. Sharfstein, Steven. [DNLM: 1. Com-
munity mental health services. WM30 N397]
RA790.N355   362.2'2   75-39312
ISBN 0-669-00429-4

Dedication

We dedicate this book to the founders of the moral treatment movement, the interpersonal humanistic therapy of an earlier era. May
attention paid to the lessons learned, both from the practice and
decline of moral treatment, assist us in assuring that neighborhood and
community psychiatry will survive and endure.

Contents

Foreword

Julius B. Richmond

Neighborhood psychiatry is an example of an idea whose time has arrived. While no one book can encompass a field which is so rapidly growing, this volume covers a wide range of concerns clearly and logically. Topics move through several descriptive levels — from a conceptual and historical frame of reference, through large-scale administrative problems, to the experiences with delivery systems and clinical issues at the local level — and chapters are presented from a variety of perspectives by administrators of programs, clinicians, and professional workers at all levels.

It is personally gratifying not only to see the growth of the field, but also to note the many talented people it has attracted. In 1965, those of us working to develop the national program of neighborhood health centers were a handful known to each other; now, for any one person to know all the workers in this field is not possible.

To comment only on what is good in this new field and what is covered in this volume, however, is not sufficient. We should also discuss areas that require increased attention in the future. One such broad area deserving more emphasis and study is that of the societal changes of the last two decades. I will briefly discuss some aspects of these changes as they provide a critical context for the work described in this book.

The increased visibility of poor people is one such a change. This has occurred as a consequence, in part, of the tremendous migration of large numbers of the poor from rural to urban poverty, and the prominence of their help-lessness and hopelessness has resulted in our having to face a range of human problems more directly. This represents an important transformation in our society. When people of low income were thinly distributed in rural areas, their problems were no less real, but they were much less obvious because so much less visible, and their oppression minimized their potential and social action. These are issues to which Dr. Pierce rightly draws attention in his commentary. The movement of people from rural to urban areas and the frustration, anger, and violence which became linked to their sense of helplessness and hopeless-ness were associated with a civil rights movement born in no small measure out of the slowness of the pace of school integration following the 1954 Supreme Court decision.

I emphasize the social issues since many of our aspirations to deliver more and better services are hampered by our failure to deal with these basic problems of racism, poverty, and inequality, as Dr. Ewalt notes in his commentary. Without better incomes, better housing, and better nutrition, the circumstances of

the poor will not change and the developmental attrition their children suffer
will not be overcome.

These are not issues for the poor alone, however. Problems in the sociology
of medical care or its broader delivery context, of access to care, equality of
treatment, and quality of service are matters forcing themselves upon the attention of persons of all income levels. Thus two forces for change have come to
have at least one point of convergence: the development of equal access to high
quality services for all. This may mean that the day of programs segregated by
economic levels — programs for the poor — will soon be over. But inherent in
this prospect is a paradox: If we are striving for *neighborhood* psychiatric services, or indeed if we are talking about *neighborhood* health services, or if we are
talking about *neighborhood* human services, it is anomalous to think services
will not be segregated by income level. How can we have neighborhood services
that are not segregated when we have not solved the problems related to segregated housing and income? The importance of focusing upon these social and
economic issues — underlying issues — is worth emphasizing if we are going to
have an integrated service system at the neighborhood level. The alternative is
to find ourselves twenty years later (as is the case in school integration twenty
years after the Supreme Court decision) trying to solve, the basic problems of
integrated services by focusing on busing people from one service center to
another rather than facing up to the integration of neighborhoods.

A second social issue which may merit increased attention in the future deals
with advocacy for better services. We have not been without advocates in the
past; indeed, at the turn of the century, people such as Jane Addams and her
associates, the Abbott sisters, the Florence Kelleys, the Dr. Alice Hamiltons,
and a host of others were charismatic advocates for all kinds of human services.
The settlement house movement centered around them.

The concept of individual advocacy seems now to have gone out of style,
perhaps because of the increasing complexity of life in this country. One of the
things with which we are now struggling is how to institutionlize this kind of
advocacy. Some of us floated this notion in the final report of the Joint Commission on Mental Health of Children and it gained greater currency in the 1970
White House Conference on Children. Understandably, concern has grown that
it is now assuming certain bureaucratic tendencies, and its original intention is
often misunderstood. Those of us who supported the idea at the national level
intended that advocacy be simply what the word means in its Anglo-Saxon
sense — that is, a form of generating support. One thing is clear: effective
advocates, must operate in areas other than only agencies and programs.

A third broad issue at this time involves the role of national health insurance
as a potential service-financing mechanism and as a force for improving services.
We have heard a great deal about the losses of support from public sources for
our various programs. I think it fair and nonpolitical to say that no one, even
in the wildest fantasy, even in greatest despair, dreamed of the kinds of

precipitous cuts that have been imposed on a variety of human service programs. It is small wonder that we are somewhat in disarray, and consequently, we are preoccupied with the immediacy of our funding problems. But it is important that we take a somewhat longer look toward the future. When (the issue is no longer "if") we develop a national health insurance program, how can we assure that provisions will be included for making possible a solid, predictable, continuing base of support for health and mental health services at the neighborhood level? This assurance would mark a sharp change from the unreliability and unpredictability with which we have lived in the past.

When national health insurance comes to pass, then, we need to be prepared to apply funding to the development of a continuing base of support so that we will not be subjected to year-to-year financing crises. Such legislation should of course incorporate provisions for prepayment rather than exclusively for fee-for-service financing, and also for making funds available to groups at the local community and neighborhood level. This will involve a good deal of creativity in devising the legislation. However, as a result of our experience with Medicare and Medicaid, we have learned a great deal about why it is important to avoid simply putting more money into an unchanged delivery system. The reasons we are having many difficulties in the financing of health services in this country at the present is that in enacting the Title XVIII and XIX Amendments to the Social Security Act, we dealt only with the financing mechanism. We made it possible to put endless sums of money into the system without incorporating mechanisms for changing the delivery of services to effect greater equity and quality. This proves an old point — that simply putting more money into an old system does not ensure that more or better services result.

The licensed health professionals have a special responsibility in this regard. In the health and mental health fields, they enjoy a monopoly; no one else is permitted to deliver the services they have the responsibility to deliver. The courts have ruled that while the licensed professions do enjoy a monopoly, they do not enjoy special privilege. The day may well be coming when the professions will be pressed to provide equal access to all population groups in an organized way. I can envision class action suits in which not only the commissioner of health or mental health but the licensed professions, through their professional association, may be called to an accounting and may be directed to submit plans whereby their services are more equitably distributed.

A related issue about which a good deal is written in this volume concerns the integration of services; the obverse of integration, of course, is fragmentation. When we express concern about integrating services, we are saying that in this country we have gone down the road of fragmentation toward categorical services far beyond the point of productivity. In fact, one might even say that if one wanted to ensure that comprehensive, family services were not going to be delivered, one would set things up in the fragmented fashion we have — category after category, whether by age group, disease group, sickness or health — so that much of our efforts are expended chasing our tails in our local communities. Indeed, local citizens sitting on the multiple boards and committees are overworked. By the time they sit on councils for the mentally retarded, mental health, maternal and infant care, child abuse services, comprehensive health planning, as well as for the many voluntary agencies, they are worn out. Until we come to terms with developing an integrated, comprehensive service system, we are not going to be as productive as we ought to be.

Integration of our present fragmented system represents one of the next major creative efforts in developing human services, and is discussed in a number of chapters in this volume. Although we will need to look at alternatives, I am concerned that we sometimes take refuge in our pluralism to the point of avoiding choices. We can retain pluralism even though we narrow the alternatives and choices. The truly creative and imaginative developments will come about by taking a position, based on experience and conviction, because we will have identified a functional, operational approach that will meet the needs of people in a community. What I suggest is that we not avoid taking a position because we are so concerned about having so many alternatives that we end up with no major commitments at all.

Of the many things that pleases me about this book, one is the increasing sophistication concerning professional roles. In connection with social action, for example, the contributors to this volume make clear that the day of the professional mental health worker acting as a community organizer, attempting to solve all the social problems in the community, is past. We are beyond that — we have learned through experience. I think that we are defining our roles more clearly and learning to work with each other more effectively. I cannot help but quote from a paper on the question of interdisciplinary activity written some years ago by Justice Felix Frankfurter: "The need for breaking down sterilizing departmentalization has been widely felt. Unfortunately, however, the too frequent way of doing it has been wittily, but not too unfairly described as a cross-sterilization of the social sciences. That is a tendency by which a difficult problem, say of the law, is solved by relying on a dubious truth in some other field."[1] We have begun to learn that as we engage in interdisciplinary activities, we need to bring back to our own discipline a clearer knowledge of *our* role and of what it is *we* can do more effectively in our own disciplines.

As I look to the future, I anticipate a great expansion of the public-private partnership about which much is written in this book. Large public agencies have serious difficulties in developing the kinds of flexibility of service delivery that they wish to have and that communities are coming to expect. On the other hand, private agencies are by no means without their own sets of rigidities. As we talk about research, evaluation, and accountability, private agencies will need to become much more flexible and open. They cannot engage in self-fulfilling prophecies which claim that because they are private and voluntary, they are necessarily better. Public agencies are not without creative innovative leadership.

Instead, many are lacking in the capacity to translate good ideas into action. We need some demonstrations of how this can be accomplished in a more effective manner. I trust we will see much more collaboration between public and private agencies, particularly through the development of contractual relationships.

The final societal issue that bears mentioning is the importance this volume attaches to a focus on the family and on the social nexus within which the family lives. Our social psychologists tell us that it is our incapacity to deal with family change and changes in family structure that is at the heart of some of our social problems. When we talk about neighborhoods and community, what we are talking about is life in the small society in which people live and work. It is this link of social nexus and service delivery that is the strength, but also the very difficult challenge, of neighborhood psychiatry — indeed of neighborhood delivery of services in general.

In closing, let me add a word of appreciation and congratulations to Drs. Macht, Scherl, and Sharfstein. They have gathered within one volume a set of vigorous chapters dealing with issues at the forefront of mental health practice today. Their book, of course, is just a beginning — an exploration of a new field and at the same time a foundation upon which others can build. The contributing authors offering their experience are pioneers who share with us their ideas — their successes and also their failures. From this volume, one can learn a great deal about what has been done and also about what remains to be done.

Reference

1. Frankfurter, F. Special Introduction in: *The Aims of Education*, Whitehead, A.N. New York: Mentor Books, 1949.

Preface

The editors of this volume were asked recently to comment on the progress of "neighborhood psychiatry" in the light of the National Health Insurance legislation now pending. Reflection on the question impressed us anew with the slow but steady movement of mental health services into a variety of neighborhood-based settings over the first half of this decade. This has occurred despite the major fiscal problems presently facing every type of program development or expansion. Not only has neighborhood psychiatry managed to endure, but new techniques, conceptualizations, and attempts at training and evaluation have grown.

However, if the neighborhood movement is to continue to thrive, the scientific literature must begin to catch up with the level of actual practice and with the importance of the public policy directions outlined in some of the chapters that follow. Opportunities are increasingly required for mental health professionals, planners, consumers, and policymakers to share their thinking and experience with regard to neighborhood mental health services.

This volume has been prepared in part as a result of our view of the need of this field for professional literature, and is written for those interested in newly developing areas in mental health. It defines the field of neighborhood psychiatry as one in which the range of clinical and community mental health functions are practiced within discrete, natural sociopolitical and geographic areas or neighborhoods. It is our hope that this book will serve to delineate where we are at present and where we may be headed. We hope it will stimulate and contribute to the work of others and will aid in turning attention to issues of service delivery as matters of serious scientific and professional interest. In a more practical vein, issues of neighborhood work have become critical to those interested in moving from an institution-based service system to a community-based one. Aftercare planning and follow-up of the increasing number of former hospital patients who seek care and support from their own neighborhoods has become a critical issue for states and localities and increasingly the neighborhood with its support systems and caregivers is being recognized as a context for the care of these long-term patients.

The book, then, grew out of the need of those involved in the field to share their experiences. Amongst the authors of individual chapters are many of the founders of neighborhood psychiatry and thus a spectrum of points of view is included with regard to mental health service delivery. It is not a handbook, as such, nor is it designed to focus only on issues of clinical practice. Instead, its central theme relates to the organization and delivery of mental health services (for adults, children, and families) in the context of current theoretical understanding and program experience in the area of comprehensive health and human services, particularly at the neighborhood level. However, the reader will find

ample program and case material in many of the chapters which give a real
sense of the actual work and experience of neighborhood practitioners. Allied
issues — research and training, for example — are included as they bear on
the central theme.

The book begins with a section devoted to matters of background and perspective in order to set the context for neighborhood psychiatry, and then
moves to the core issue of program models for organization and delivery of
mental health services at the neighborhood level. Issues of research and training
are considered next. The book closes with an epilogue chapter which considers
recent federal and state public policy initiatives that reflect the context for and
the impact of neighborhood psychiatry and which presents a view of the future
of this new field of theory and practice. This view includes matters such as the
neighborhood-based care of former state hospital patients, prevention, program
evaluation, public education, and critical issues of neighborhood and community
development.

The volume contains original chapters by various authors as well as chapters
and commentary by the editors. Some of the material is expanded and updated
from papers presented at a national three-day conference held at the Massachusetts Institute of Technology in June of 1973. It was cosponsored by the Center
for Neighborhood Mental Health Services Research and Training, Massachusetts
Department of Mental Health, Massachusetts Department of Public Health,
Massachusetts Institute of Technology, the Cambridge Hospital, Cambridge-
Somerville Mental Health and Retardation Center, and the Massachusetts League
of Neighborhood Health Centers. Over 500 people attended the conference in
which over 50 practitioners participated. The book is not a proceedings of the
conference however. Rather, it is an attempt to build upon concepts and papers
first presented at that time in order to provide an overview of the new field of
neighborhood psychiatry. This volume of course goes far beyond where the
field was in 1973. While some chapters are based on material prepared for the
conference, others were written exclusively for this volume.

A book such as this is prepared only with the diligent work and support of
many people. The editors want to thank, in particular, the various contributing
authors, as well as our senior editorial assistants, Donna M. Foley, Mardee B.
Carter, and Dale Chadwick, and our editorial assistants, Susan Finn and Judith
Salerno. They all added immeasurably to the final product and made possible
its completion through their patience, diligence, and especially their good humor.
Lois Macht has been a constant source of encouragement and support for these
efforts and has also assisted in the review of the manuscript; without her it
would not have been possible. Gerald Caplan, M.D., provided advice and support
in the early planning. Dean William M. Capron of the Kennedy School of
Government at Harvard and the National Institute of Mental Health permitted
time and support for one of the editors to assist in the editing. However this

volume does not necessarily represent the official position of the NIMH. John E. Mack, M.D., and Robert C. Reid, M.D., provided encouragement and support and allowed for the time of another of the editors to complete the work. The book represents the views of the authors and editors alone, however, and not the official policy of the National Institute of Mental Health or any of the other organizations with which the editors or contributing authors are affiliated. Finally, the authors gratefully acknowledge their debt to Julius B. Richmond, M.D., who has been a resilient source of encouragement, support, and wisdom.

October, 1976   *Lee B. Macht*
Boston, Massachusetts   *Donald J. Scherl*
                                                         Steven Sharfstein

Part I

Neighborhood Psychiatry: Background Issues and Perspectives

Introduction

This section includes chapters which set the context from which neighborhood psychiatry arose and within which it must now be practiced. The several authors sketch the history, organization, policy, and critical practical and conceptual aspects of the field. As an introduction, these papers, dealing with a broad spectrum of topics, provide a comprehensive overview of the field — its dimensions and relationships. This section attempts to delineate issues which form the backdrop for subsequent sections covering various specific aspects of neighborhood psychiatry in detail.

The chapter by Macht describes the historical roots of neighborhood psychiatry and outlines alternative patterns of practice and currently pressing issues in neighborhood work. Ewalt, in his commentary, points to some of the particular pitfalls, dangers, and excesses of which neighborhood mental health workers must beware. Pierce comments, in turn, on the critical interrelationship of neighborhood practice and the fight of oppressed groups for greater power and freedom.

The section continues with Scherl's description of the evolving human services field. He emphasizes the intimate link of neighborhood psychiatry to other concurrent attempts to provide comprehensive services on a local basis and to the organizational structures which have evolved to foster these efforts. He describes the discontents which gave impetus to the human services movement and the limitations of the movement in its own right and as it bears upon mental health services. This context becomes important as an introduction to the section on program models, since state and national organizational planning has a clear impact on neighborhood practice.

As Scherl examines the governmental and organizational context, Naparstek and Haskell provide a critical discussion of neighborhood services viewed from the vantage point of the urban policy specialist. They deal with issues of decentralization of government and of building a neighborhood infrastructure based upon citizen participation. They also deal in a substantive fashion with issues of ethnicity and mental health service delivery broadening some of the material presented in the chapter by Macht which begins Part I. Their chapter highlights the dilemmas of this evolving social system context for neighborhood practitioners attempting to function within it.

The section concludes with a chapter by Walsh and Bicknell which traces the evolution, principles, failings, successes, and underlying premises of the neighborhood health center. Since much of neighborhood psychiatry is practiced in such settings, an understanding of the health centers is essential to what follows.

Overall, then, this section is a broad-based introduction to the field from a number of different perspectives to provide the reader with an understanding of the issues and background necessary for appreciating neighborhood psychiatric programs, research, and training matters as they evolved.

1 An Introduction to the Field

Lee B. Macht

Although neighborhood services have their roots in even the earliest days of American psychiatry, Adolph Meyer must be credited with having dreamed the dream in 1915 which has come to fruition in our time:

However much of a dreamer I may be, I pride myself on having seen a good many of my dreams come true. Can you see the ward or district organization with a district center with reasonably accurate records of the facts needed for orderly work? Among the officers a district health officer, a district school committee and a district improvement and recreation committee, a tangible expression of what the district stands for . . . ? I long to get the means and the privilege of trying a few mental hygiene districts, no doubt best shaped, as things are now subdivided, so as to have the school of the district as the center of attention with a specially trained physician and two or three helpers living in the district, without any trumpets and without legislation; as far as possible inconspicuous, but charged to obtain the friendship and cooperation of the teachers, the district workers of various charity organizations and the physicians and ministers of the region. They would have to know their districts as a social fabric and they can do so if their districts are not too large; they must become helpers of individuals and families when they are in a mood to listen.[1]

Meyer was one of the original dreamers of neighborhood psychiatry; present practitioners inherit his dream.

We practice when several historical and current factors allow us to work in neighborhood settings. The purpose of this chapter is to provide an introduction to the field by briefly locating some of the roots of this new development in the delivery of mental health services and then examining our legacy, looking briefly at program models and issues in neighborhood psychiatry. This chapter provides a backdrop in broad brush strokes for the chapters which follow indicating where we have been and where we currently are in this field.

Historical Perspective

We may define neighborhood psychiatry in a preliminary fashion, as mental health work within an identifiable geographic, psychosocial, and sociopolitical area or neighborhood (including mental health practice within a particular facility or facilities such as neighborhood health and multiservice centers, as well as with neighborhood organizations and networks). The particular kind of practice may

5

include direct clinical services for children and adults, consultation and collaboration with other caregivers, and the development of and work with social networks in the neighborhood. Looked at from this perspective, several historical roots of neighborhood psychiatry are visible. More detailed historical treatments from other perspectives may be found elsewhere [2,3].

First, is the long history of the movement of services closer to where people live and work. Although the early state hospitals did have community linkages [4], Jarvis in his 1855 report, *Insanity and Idiocy in Massachusetts: A Report of the Commission on Lunacy* [5], documented that psychiatric facilities (then state mental hospitals) were used most by people who resided in areas surrounding the hospital or where transportation routes existed. He, together with Meyer fifty years later, strongly advocated bringing facilities closer to "the people who ought to use them." Except for some practice in general hospitals (e.g., Benjamin Rush at the Pennsylvania Hospital in the mid-eighteenth century), the practice of public psychiatry remained largely state-hospital based until the development of psychopathic hospitals in the early part of this century. This was followed by major developments in the area of public outpatient psychiatric clinics, child guidance clinics, and satellite clinics of hospitals during the second and third decades of this century [3].

Although Caplan described a relatively early experiment (1951) with the delivery of mental health services in neighborhood centers in Jerusalem [6], a large-scale opportunity was not present in this country until 1963 for developing comprehensive community-based mental health programs. In 1963 Congress enacted the Community Mental Health Centers Act, followed by the Economic Opportunity Act of 1964. The confluence of the community mental health movement and the "war on poverty" brought about a number of important developments in the history of the delivery of mental health services. The decade of the sixties set in motion policies which brought about the development of mental health services based in the community simultaneously with neighborhood health and multiservice centers. Programs such as OEO's Job Corps began to demonstrate that mental health services could be effectively integrated into comprehensive health services. Not until the late sixties, however, and early in the present decade did these developments begin to coalesce. Mental health centers developed increased linkages with neighborhood facilities, mental health became a component of comprehensive health programs, and large-scale planning for the integration of all human services at various organizational levels was initiated. Subsequent chapters deal with many of the issues raised by these developments.

A second historical root is inherent in the close link between medicine and psychiatry. From the standpoint of service delivery, the development of general hospital psychiatry had great bearing on neighborhood psychiatry practice. Beginning with the appointment of Benjamin Rush, one of the founders of American psychiatry, to the staff of the Pennsylvania Hospital in 1765, psychiatric practice became part of the development of general health services as they have continued to grow in this century. Concurrent developments of community medicine and community mental health in the 1960s represent further extensions of efforts to improve the delivery of health services. These trends converge with the development of comprehensive neighborhood services and neighborhood-based mental health services during this time period.

A third root is found in the marriage of psychiatry and social work. Our present perspective assumes that conjoint work in these two fields is necessary in order to provide services. However, clear recognition of the importance of the social setting and social history for psychiatry did not occur until this century, with the work of Meyer, Harry Stack Sullivan, and others. Meyer, for example, regularly employed his wife, a social worker, to obtain socioenvironmental data about his patients. The efforts of Elmer Southard, a psychiatrist, and Mary Jarrett, a social worker, culminated in their 1922 volume, *The Kingdom of Evils* [7], which reflected the importance of the collaboration between these two fields in dealing with mental health problems. The mental hygiene, child guidance, and orthopsychiatry movements furthered close working relationships between these two disciplines in the 1920s and 1930s. This root, like the others had its own interesting historical development for the area of neighborhood mental health: early settlement house work and other neighborhood programs provided the settings wherein social workers were in fact the first mental health workers focused on the neighborhood. Southard and Jarrett in 1922 gave a preview of the present scene when they made what was then a revolutionary statement:

As the horizons of medicine widen, it is conceivable that the hospital of the future may be a social institution, administered by men of sociological-medical training. The community, no doubt, will more and more demand that the hospital treat the whole man, that the treatment of disease aim at complete social adjustment, and that the hospital go outside its walls to prevent disease.[7]

A fourth root lies in the enormous expansion of mental health manpower which has taken place since World War II. The movement of new professionals, especially nurses, into the field during the 1960s has helped to provide adequate manpower to staff active treatment inpatient facilities. New manpower both allows and forces us to turn more attention to ambulatory care facilities, which many inpatient units can now be. The development of psychiatric nursing with a community focus — similar to that of public health nursing — has proven vital to the development of neighborhood services.

A fifth root lies in the development of clinical psychiatry to the point where many conditions can be treated on an ambulatory basis or with relatively brief hospitalizations. Improvements in psychological, social, and somatic therapies during this century have highlighted the entire area of ambulatory care. Experience in military psychiatry during World War I and subsequent wars has demonstrated the clinical importance of treating people close to or within their usual social networks. The usefulness of returning patients to these networks and support systems in order to prevent the institutionalization and dependency resulting from chronic hospitalization has also been demonstrated. Neighborhood services have become bases for aftercare as well as for primary clinical practice. As psychiatric care has improved, we have been faced with the same dilemma as our medical colleagues — how best to deliver what we know to those who need our services. Neighborhood psychiatry as part of our caregiving system is an important new addition.

A sixth historical root is found in the development of citizen participation. In the mental health field, this evolved from the earlier work of reformers of the late nineteenth and early twentieth centuries, such as Dorothea Dix and Clifford Beers. These citizen leaders shaped many trends from the mental hygiene movement through the development of mental health associations, to the current era of various advocacy groups in the field. Citizen participation, carried into the experience of the war on poverty and the community mental health centers movement, in turn, became an important factor in shaping the health care delivery system through such mechanisms as community boards and consumer representation in the planning process. Consumers have served to highlight the importance of neighborhood-based services.

A seventh root, and the final one to be described here, lies in the development of practical and theoretical elements of community psychiatry. The past twenty years have seen major developments in population-centered approaches matched by theoretical ideas in social psychiatry and social systems theory. Advances in our thinking about prevention, the influence of social and environmental factors in mental health and illness, as well as advances in consultation and collaboration theory and technique, and the beginnings of a psychiatric epidemiology, provide important scientific and theoretical bases for neighborhood psychiatry.

This brief overview of the historical roots of neighborhood psychiatry work brings us to a consideration of the state of the field today. An outline of the major programmatic and conceptual issues which emerge as the legacy of neighborhood psychiatry follows.

The Practice of Neighborhood Psychiatry

Neighborhood psychiatry is practiced in a number of different contexts involving various patterns of service delivery that may be classified as: solo neighborhood mental health delivery (where mental health workers operate directly in neighborhoods or within storefronts, satellites, mobile vans, or other neighborhood bases), and mental health services within comprehensive neighborhood health or human service centers [2].

In the latter settings, mental health workers work within broader health and social service programs available in a neighborhood. Several patterns have emerged within this category. In one, the mental health worker serves as a consultant; no direct service is provided but consultation to primary caregivers is the mode of operation. In the second pattern, the mental health service works in isolation within a neighborhood health center — a mental health service existing within a more comprehensive neighborhood service center but not integrated with other services. In a third, the mental health service is an integral part of a comprehensive health center: mental health workers become members of the overall staff and integral partners of comprehensive care teams. A final pattern consists of the mental health service as an integral part of a comprehensive center with a mental health worker in a position of executive responsibility within the organization. In this model, the mental health worker has overall clinical and planning authority within the comprehensive center and works to integrate the range of services, including mental health.

Within each of these patterns, except that of pure consultation, the range of direct treatment and indirect techniques used by the mental health worker includes consultation, coordination, education, and collaboration. In addition, the opportunity exists to work on social and environmental factors with neighborhood residents. Neighborhood practice, though similar to other mental health work, is distinctly different, bringing with it a keener sense of the patient's life situation. It not only clearly highlights the importance of a variety of caregiving systems in helping people solve problems, but presents the practical need for integration of services. When practicing in a neighborhood, the mental health worker also comes to appreciate the strengths, talents, and struggles of people living in the neighborhood.

For example, the clinical situation of a 40-year-old, depressed mother of two who recently lost a third child in an auto accident outside the housing project where she lives, has a more palpable reality for the worker when seen in the neighborhood against the environmental backdrop of fear and chaos, single-parent families, poor housing, and lack of adequate recreational facilities for children. The clinician in neighborhood practice must confront these realities in a different way than when he sees a similar patient in a hospital office. Interventions must therefore be geared to that aspect of a patient's life — be it internal or external — where it makes the most sense to attempt a therapeutic change. The assessment of this issue and techniques for achieving appropriate ends require the attention of the neighborhood mental health worker at yet another level (described further elsewhere [8]).

To provide another illustration, the neighborhood mental health practitioner sees a different aspect of an otherwise ordinary mental health issue when he recognizes that a chronic schizophrenic patient in acute exacerbation is only one of many acutely distressed people in a housing project from which rent control has just been removed. A number of the patient's neighbors have come to the neighborhood health center with depression, anxiety, and psychophysiological symptoms; they feel helpless, hopeless, and furious [8]. The practitioner witnesses tenant meetings where groups of neighbors unite to take action, regain some control over their lives, and demonstrate to themselves that they can influence what happens; he is forced to ponder which has been more important in alleviating distress: individual ministrations to patients or the larger-scale intervention of social action. The practitioner must therefore also consider possibilities of intervention through social networks, portions of the neighborhood and larger subsystems, as well as with individuals and families.

The practitioner can also observe the psychological growth and increase in self-esteem of neighborhood residents who serve on the board of a center or work as caregivers within it. Firsthand experience emphasizes that mental health practice in the neighborhood inevitably involves collaboration with general health workers, welfare and neighborhood workers, clergy, police, housing, recreation, and legal staff, as well as many other caregivers, and these people are crucial in preventive interventions on behalf of the patients and neighborhood people. The integration of human services thus becomes more than theory and distant planning; instead, it is a reality of day-to-day work growing out of the neighborhood context. The neighborhood and its internal human service systems are the most fruitful common pathway for integrating service delivery.

Issues

We now turn to some issues raised by the phenomenology of neighborhood psychiatry which subsequent chapters will address in greater depth. First, why do mental health practitioners work in neighborhoods? The reasons are more than the important and often-stated one of physical proximity. While it is important to bring services closer to people if they are to be utilized effectively, other reasons for this work include the fact that local facilities are often seen as belonging to the neighborhood and part of it, not distant and alien like a hospital or mental health clinic. This is especially true in facilities with active neighborhood boards and workers from the neighborhood. Further, such a facility can more readily respond to the needs of neighborhood residents as they define those needs since the local center is an integral part of the socio-cultural-political matrix — the life processes of the neighborhood. Access is also available to other caregivers, to the natural institutions and systems of the neighborhood, to groups of people residing in close proximity, and to the informal as well as formal support systems which help people in distress.

A second issue relates to the concept of outreach and satellite clinics. Leopold and Kissick [9] have dealt with this issue as has English [9]. However, precisely because a neighborhood facility can become the primary caregiving nexus, the concept of neighborhood services as mainly "outreach" or "satellite" has outlived its usefulness. We must, rather, view these services as integral and primary components of a rational caregiving system in mental health. They are the front line; the mental health center or hospital is specialized backup, primarily to provide inpatient services and a choice of a place to obtain care for those who (for reasons of confidentiality or other factors) prefer to go to a central rather than a neighborhood facility [10]. In the long-term development of mental health services, I would suggest that the community mental health center, developed in the sixties and emphasized as the major caregiving institution, will prove to be transitional as we advance to more truly community-based services. Neighborhood psychiatry can provide these services more effectively because neighborhood centers are more integral community organizations than are centralized mental health centers.

A third issue relates to the need for improved research and evaluation in mental health services delivery. The question is whether we can develop a methodology for evaluating theoretical assumptions and testable hypotheses in this field. We are only in the earliest phases of this task but must move forward rapidly to design more rational systems of care in mental health. In the area of neighborhood mental health, we need to know, minimally, such things as: who uses these programs and why; whether they are more "effective" (as defined by the neighborhood, the caregivers, and other accountability structures) than other ways of delivering care; their cost compared to that of other systems; the effects of integrating services; whether primary prevention is possible through neighborhood or any other types of services; and how mental health workers satisfy or fail to satisfy the needs of neighborhood people.

A fourth issue concerns integration of services. We need to address ourselves to such questions as when service integration is useful (and why) and when separation of mental health services might be preferable. For example, for many low-income people, mental health is of low priority; in order to reach the people who need care, it makes sense to integrate mental health services with job training, general health, education, welfare, and other human services. Mental health services may become more responsive to mainstream needs if they are integrated with other services which are seen as high priority. Further, some evidence [8] indicates that integrating human services parallels early caregiving systems in the human life cycle, such as the early parent-child relationship in which the child turns to a parent to provide the range of necessary human needs. This model may have implications for both the kind of human service systems people utilize most readily and for the patterns of integrated care which must be devised.

We must also examine the losses to the mental health professions that come from integration. Is our training in the various mental health fields compromised when no longer limited to a categorical problem? Are the possibilities for development of our own science compromised by integration? My own view is that the opportunities for education in the various mental health disciplines will be greatly enhanced in multiservice settings providing increased opportunities for basic clinical as well as community mental health training. Our science will profit in these new settings which provide rich opportunities for different kinds of clinical experience as well as for operational program research which can advance scientific progress in mental health.

Is funding for mental health services and programs endangered when they are no longer separately identifiable? Mental health planners and workers will have to fight vigorously for financial support in integrated service systems and mental health professionals will have to take leadership roles within these programs, at various levels, to ensure that the mental health services receive a proper share of the limited finances for human services. However, we must also acknowledge that funds for general health, welfare, education, and housing are important for an effective mental health effort, and that categorical support for mental health programs may not be the only way in which mental health related funds can be put to good use.

A fifth issue asks whether neighborhood psychiatry is a separately identifiable field and if so, what kinds of theories can be developed for it, and upon what other theoretical points of view does it depend? The neighborhood context clearly delineates neighborhood psychiatry as a distinct type of mental health practice. It extends clinical practice to include more active engagement with the realities of the patient's daily life in the patient's home setting and incorporates other caregivers, including family and neighbors, into a network. From the standpoint of theory, this kind of work draws upon individual psychodynamic, group dynamic, mental health consultation, and social systems theories. It is involved with the interface of individual and social psychology. As an area of specialized concern, neighborhood psychiatry must move to develop its own theories of interaction between the individual and his surroundings (interpersonal and physical) and particularly its own theories of intervention.

A sixth issue focuses on whether lessons learned from work in low-income neighborhoods, where the majority of neighborhood facilities exist, can be applied to middle-class, suburban, and rural areas. While patterns of services vary according to individual and population styles and needs, models of neighborhood psychiatry are applicable outside the inner city. Such models now apply to group practices, health maintenance organizations, small town and rural service networks.

A seventh issue concerns education and training in neighborhood psychiatry. We must build good clinical training programs which hopefully can deal with the importance of social and environmental as well as intrapsychic, developmental, and familial factors. We must go further in this field to provide training in how to work with and within the new forms through which services are being delivered and must teach the techniques and theories of consultation, coordination, collaboration, social action, and community organization and development.

An eighth and final issue relates to the problems, dilemmas, and limitations of neighborhood practice. Certainly the problem of confidentiality is major in neighborhood work and must be considered carefully; so too must the dilemma of residents who work in their own neighborhoods. Problems of funding for neighborhood psychiatry are major and threaten to impede progress. We must look to reimbursement, health insurance, revenue sharing, health maintenance organizations, and possibilities of shifting staff from funded central mental health centers and state hospitals to front-line facilities. Major and difficult decisions face policy makers, legislators, administrators, clinicians, and citizens in moving from a demonstration phase to major program implementation in neighborhood mental health. We must also deal with our own limitations in effecting major changes in the quality of life in the neighborhoods where we work and must question our ability to provide meaningful services in neighborhoods. The final chapter of this volume also addresses these issues further. We share with the mental health field in general the question of whether neighborhood psychiatry – or any other form of practice in the profession – can effect the incidence and prevalence of mental illness.

References

1. Meyer, A. "Where should we attack the problem of the prevention of mental defect and mental disease?" *The Collected Papers of Adolph Meyer.* E.E. Winters (ed.) Baltimore: Johns Hopkins Press, 1952.
2. Macht, L.B. "Neighborhood Psychiatry." *Psychiatric Annals, 4*:9, September, 1974.
3. Ewalt, J.R. and Ewalt, P.L. "History of the Community Psychiatry Movement." *American Journal of Psychiatry, 126*: 43-53, 1969.
4. Caplan, R.B. *Psychiatry and the Community in Nineteenth Century America.* Basic Books, Inc.: New York, 1969.
5. Jarvis, E. "Insanity and Idiocy in Massachusetts: Report of the Commission on Lunacy", 1855. Cambridge: Harvard University Press, 1971.
6. Caplan, G. "A Public Health Approach to Child Psychiatry". *Mental Hygiene,* XXXV: 235-249, 1951.
7. Southard, E.E. and Jarrett, M.C. *The Kingdom of Evils.* New York: MacMillan Co., 1922.
8. Scherl, D.J., Macht, L.B., and Sharfstein, S. "Beyond the Mental Health Center: Neighborhood Psychiatry". Monograph. In preparation.
9. Leopold, R.L. and Kissick, W.L. "A Community Mental Health Center, Regional Medical Programs, and Joint Planning." *American Journal of Psychiatry* 126:1718-26 June 1970.

10. Macht, L.B. "Beyond the Mental Health Center: Planning for a Community of Neighborhoods". *Psychiatric Annals,* 5: 7, July, 1975.

2

Commentaries on Neighborhood Psychiatry

Jack R. Ewalt and *Chester M. Pierce*

Commentary by Jack R. Ewalt

As early as 1912, Adolph Meyer and the then Commissioner of Mental Health in Massachusetts, Dr. Copp, advocated the formation of district mental health centers. Despite many problems and a few solutions, the dream has continued to grow. Since it is a movement with which I have great sympathy, I would like to go beyond talking about mental health programs and their advantages, and raise three questions that keep recurring to me. I raise them because I feel they are important enough to require answers, although I have none at the present time.

The first deals with the problem of psychiatry moving so far out into the community that it begins to deal with patients suffering in relation to real rather than irrational situations. I question the morality, the good sense, or the usefulness of diagnosing as a psychiatric problem the depressed, angry, and discouraged mother with a number of children who lives in poverty in the slums. It seems to me that such a person who is depressed, paranoid, angry, and perhaps militant is reacting rationally to a real-life situation. Her happy neighbor, hoping for a better life in the hereafter, who brings her sad friend to the clinic for help is probably the one reacting irrationally.

Caution in our thinking and modification of our practices are required to "treat" the uncomfortable, suffering, but normal person with personal support, empathy, and perhaps medication, together with encouragement to participate in social efforts and pressures to better his or her life. Spending time in individual, group, or family therapy exploring the dynamics of the depression or paranoia of such a person is fatuous. People in these situations need help in terms of social not personal change, and as citizens we should help them to bring that change about. However, the time of highly trained therapists is better spent on persons reacting irrationally, though with similar symptomatology, to a more standard set of internal and social stresses, such as married life, the need to work, the pressures of upward mobility, political chicanery, and so forth.

A second worrisome feature deserving emphasis concerns the confidentiality of the patient's name, record, and history. Increasingly, insurance companies, welfare departments, and other agencies are demanding detailed personal and medical information (sometimes running to pages) about the individuals who come to them for some type of income assistance or health care support. Providing such information violates the confidence the patient expects both morally

15

and legally from medical institutions and practitioners. Withholding the information, however, means the person may not be granted the support needed. This situation raises the serious question of whether privacy in personal and medical matters has become a luxury dependent upon income level. Identifying the patient by a code number, together with a statement by the caring physician that the patient is or is not disabled, should be sufficient. The granting agency could then consult with the physician chosen by the insurance company or welfare department to validate the patient's claim for care. At present, such procedures will not be accepted as a basis for payment.

The third category of concern is a little thorny and is directly related to the movement of patient care resources into the neighborhood or family life center. An important and viable part of this process is the pressure to have patients move from state hospitals back into the neighborhoods. Like mother love, the idea on superficial consideration is a great one, but, like mother love, cases vary tremendously. For some patients, movement back into the real world offers enormous stimulation and help. But it is very important that meaningful and concerned persons be available and ready to assist the patient in this rehabilitation program. To abandon the patient to the loneliness of a room in a boarding house, by whatever fancy name, without the support of a person he loves and trusts is more cruel than leaving him where he was.

Further, many patients develop attachments to personnel or other patients in the hospital community itself. One questions the humaneness of moving these patients, particularly as they reach later life; Not only does the danger exist that their long-standing psychotic condition will flare-up, but actual mortality is associated with moving older people into new settings. Both New York City and California welfare services are beginning to report problems with abuse of patients released back into communities.

I am not speaking about the large number of patients who will do better in community settings, but, rather, of the smaller number who will do much better, in my opinion, in the old system. As we become more adept in offering care to patients at or near their homes, hopefully we can expect that they will come to the attention of helping personnel earlier, that necessary, definitive therapy will be applied earlier, and as a result, that fewer patients will become chronic and develop dependence on institutions. In the meantime, however, we must be humane to the victims of age and neglect and not force them into a new stereotype. Rather, we must make an effort to study the individual's needs and try to provide beneficial services, regardless of the effects on departmental or public plans and statistics.

Commentary by Chester M. Pierce

The chapters of this book outline and define the boundaries of what should become a new, vibrant, and necessary field. We must address the knotty social and political problems that they stimulate. Discussion of neighborhood psychiatry actually addresses itself to *why* people are oppressed and *how* they are oppressed — to sociopolitical considerations. Each chapter states that psychiatry's role regarding these considerations should be defined and made operational.

From my viewpoint, the *how* of people being oppressed involves the oppressed and the oppressor being trained via cumulative microaggressions to permit, accept, and expect that the oppressed should be abused, degraded, demeaned, and devalued. In terms of both service and research, psychiatrists and other mental health workers must understand how these demeaning microaggressions are delivered. Their delivery in a subtle, ongoing, never-ending manner characterizes the relationship between the oppressor and the oppressed and ensures that the victim will maintain a forced dependency.

Why people are oppressed in our society involves racial and class considerations. Generally, the oppressed are colored (red, black, brown, yellow) and the oppression sustains their poverty. Since they are powerless in promoting an enlightened revision of custom, they remain poor and oppressed. The enlightened revision of custom is, by definition, the law. The law, and the commitment of resources to the oppressed, has been too slender to banish social injustices, the root of much emotional anguish.

The oppressed themselves will have to initiate and maintain pressures in order to ameliorate their plight. Neighborhood practitioners must aid this process. One way to do so is educative. Hopefully, the day is not too remote when every citizen will be sensitive and informed in such areas as systems analysis, demography, and propaganda. Such knowledge will allow the neighborhood to participate positively in its own defense and definition, and individual members of the neighborhood will no longer be psychologically geared to permit and expect oppression.

This book engages in an exciting task. Toward this goal, the first chapter might very well become a classic in defining what will become neighborhood psychiatry and one of the new directions in which mental health will move. It serves as a good departure point, raising incontestable points which must be pursued and resolved. The movement may seem beyond the pale of tradition to many of today's praticing professionals. I submit that the person who practiced psychiatry in 1890 would not understand the psychiatry of 1976 as practiced by those who work on Wilshire Boulevard or Fifth Avenue. By 1990, the concepts discussed in this volume may be commonplace in the practice of psychiatry, as well as other mental health disciplines.

3

Reorganization of the Human Services and the Practice of Neighborhood Psychiatry

Donald J. Scherl

The shift in emphasis of public mental health practice from the state hospital to the community mental health center and now to the neighborhood has paralleled in time a movement toward linking and integrating all of the health and social services into comprehensive systems for the delivery of care for those with special needs. Neighborhood psychiatry, as it is practiced today, must be viewed not only in the context of the natural setting of the neighborhood but also within organizational frameworks which may (or may not) be neighborhood based and are linked with, and reflective of, city, state, and national bureaucratic organizational entities. Any consideration of neighborhood psychiatry must therefore include an examination of these larger organizational contexts for service delivery. This chapter explores briefly the newly evolving human services movement as one important element with which neighborhood-based psychiatric practice must deal.

The United States has entered an era in which services for people with special needs have become a matter of increasing public concern. One element of this concern involves dissatisfaction on the part of special interest groups, providers, the press, budget experts, the judiciary, politicians, and the general public with the way in which services have been arranged and delivered. If this dissatisfaction can be said to focus on a single issue, it is that of devising a system of services for people in need which is problem-centered rather than institution- or profession-centered. The issue is how to develop an incentive system to facilitate the evolution of community and neighborhood networks which will bring categorical services together from their current state of physical, and at times conceptual, separateness.

The solution toward which the federal government, many states, and some of the larger municipalities groped in the 1960s and early 1970s involved combining governmental functions into logical and larger aggregates. The trend was to make government, at whatever level, more manageable, more rational, more adaptable and, recently, less costly. To achieve this end, over half of the states have now developed structural frameworks along lines represented by large umbrella agencies called "Human Resources" or "Human Services." From an organizational point of view, the human services agency is, in one sense, a governmental conglomerate — a holding company within which each state or city has grouped together one or another set of categorical organizational entities. To place the human services movement in some perspective, it may be useful to review several of the trends out of which it has emerged, using the health and mental health systems as examples.

Historical Perspectives

Two major discontents have coalesced to support the emergence of more comprehensively designed services for people. First has been the frustration commonly encountered when people attempt to obtain the range of services they need at any one point in time. The problems and irritations of shopping from agency to agency and from specialist to specialist, whether one pays for services directly, has insurance which does so, or depends on the government, are familiar to all. Individuals and families continue to encounter endless difficulties when their problems are not categorized in a manner which qualifies them to receive aid from a single agency or practitioner.

The historical roots from which this discontent has grown are of interest. With reference to health and mental health services, 150 years ago facilities were localized and, in one sense, comprehensive. The local jail or almshouse provided such aid as was available for the retarded, the mentally ill, the poor, and the criminal. The reform of that era saw the development of separate specialized services (health, mental health, welfare) and of increasing professionalism. For the mentally ill and the retarded, this change was marked by the development of the state hospital system and the transfer of responsibility for the mentally ill from the locality to the state [1].

At the same time, the medical subspeciality of psychiatry was developing. In the early 1900s, specialization emerged in all of the health professions. This was accelerated by advances in the natural sciences which resulted in the 1930s in the development of the medical specialty boards. Since the 1940s, specialization and subspecialization have become important elements of medical and psychiatric practice [2]. Although this has improved the quality of care immeasurably, it has led simultaneously to a fragmentation of the health care delivery system, sometimes actually making services harder for people to obtain.

Concurrent with emergence of increased specialization, the separation of psychiatry and mental health from the health and social services with which they were previously linked increased. Separate psychiatric institutions developed, making the provision of a broad range of services for the client increasingly difficult. The design of prevention programs involving interventions of both a social and a health character became more difficult since these services were no longer clustered together.

The second major area of discontent helping to give rise to the human services movement involved governmental structure and management. Over the past two decades state and local governments have increased enormously in size and responsibility. As late as the 1960s and early 1970s, however, their structure

and organization reflected, in the main, the same basic pattern that had persisted
for the prior hundred years. Bureaus, agencies, and departments were conceived,
grew, and multiplied as pressure for new functions dictated. Their growth was
random and their purpose sporadic and categorically specific. In the Commonwealth of Massachusetts, for example, the end product was several hundred
departments, boards, commissions, agencies, and authorities, each of which was
independently and separately responsible to the Governor.

Additionally, the 1960s and 1970s witnessed a rising eagerness of citizens to
be involved in the provision, direction, and monitoring of services at the various
levels of government and in the private sector. Difficulties in determining which
citizens, which services, and what kind of involvement are well known and require
no reiteration here. Clearly, however, as units of government have devised more
broadly conceived organizational frameworks, citizen groups have increasingly
desired an even stronger voice in the functional affairs of these agencies.

In many ways, state departments of mental health represent a paradigm of
government as it had evolved and of the dissatisfaction felt by many groups with
it. In many states, these departments had become enormously large bureaucracies
involving central, regional, and local offices. State hospitals for the mentally ill
and state schools for the mentally retarded existed in total or partial isolation
from evolving community alternatives. The system became dominated by paper
flow; forms generated more forms, and administrative costs rose without any
concomitant improvement in management. Decisions were made administratively in isolation from the citizens affected by them. As a result, in addition to the
traditional boards of visitors or trustees for state institutions, new entities arose
in local areas claiming to represent mental health and mental retardation interests
and formed into self-annointed or government-designated "area boards" or
"councils." This patchwork of services, advocates, and bureaucrats existed in
many states in virtual isolation from allied service systems involving social
services, public welfare, services for the physically handicapped, and so forth.
No wonder, then, the rising tide of discontent.

Problems and Opportunities

In addition to the two major dissatisfactions which coalesced to give impetus to
the human services movement, a number of other emergent concerns also looked
to the movement for a comprehensive cure. People hoped that the grouping
and integration of services under a human services umbrella agency would somehow solve the physical separation of services, devise new models for service
delivery, and ensure a high quality of service for all in need. Nothing short of
another Creation could satisfy all of these hopes. The human services movement,
then, was bound to elicit disappointment and such has been the case. It may be
useful to describe a number of separate trends which have attempted to find

expression through the human services movement, and to consider whether there are elements inherent in developing and implementing a broadly based comprehensive human service system which of necessity lead to certain dangerous misunderstandings.

*Local Services, Locally Controlled: Decentralization
and Deinstitutionalization*

The need to integrate or link services through the development of local service networks seems clear. To that end, new models of delivery — multiservice centers, community mental health centers, neighborhood health centers and others — have emerged. Each can claim authority and prerogative to coordinate and integrate services locally and, indeed, each does so. (Ironically, the more comprehensive the program becomes, the more it resembles that hardy relic of the past, the settlement house: this institution, often a product of benevolence, was a part of its neighborhood in a real and integral sense, often housing the widest imaginable array of health, social, recreational and educational programs and services.)

The decentralization of services implies that responsibility for program decisions and for development of flexible and diverse service systems and linkages must be a local responsibility under local control. A system of local service delivery subject to professional, state, and federal quality control, operating within specified guidelines, and utilizing block funding offers the hope of a framework within which the specialized (categorical) services currently existing can be made to work for, rather than against, the client. Local decision making also implies, however, that localities must be willing to accept as their own the special needs of all their citizens, including, for example, the emotionally, intellectually, and chronically impaired, the physically handicapped, the blind, the deaf, and the adult and youthful offender.

The increasing focus on the prevention of institutionalization is almost totally dependent on the development of these local service systems. Preventing clients from being sent away from their community or making their return possible (or desirable) is impossible without making available a local, comprehensive, better organized array of services. These include medical, psychological, educational, and social services; manpower training and supported work; and counseling and rehabilitation programs. All of these necessary, specialized support services must be available and ready for use as needed for each client and family. Community after community and state after state has amply demonstrated the possibility of bringing clients from institutions back into the community and in many cases of preventing their removal in the first instance. The absence of adequate local services for mental hospital patients, however, has led to reports of "dumping" patients onto the streets, into nursing homes,

* and into sleazy, single-room occupancy, hotel/rooming houses. For those who have made deinstitutionalization an ideology, the reality of what they impose upon the discharged patient, for whom the community is not prepared, seems at best outside the realm of their interest, and at worst, a deliberate creation of human misery in the name of "social change."

A second myth for those involved in the human services movement to heed is the fantasy that community-based services organized on a human services model represent something for which people have been waiting eagerly. Experience has demonstrated that this is not so. It will be a long while before the majority of citizens in any neighborhood want to care for those with special needs within their own neighborhood and on their own block. Those who have attempted to establish halfway houses for special need groups, whether for the retarded, the alcoholic, or the youthful offender are acutely aware of this situation. If there were no other reason to fully involve the community in the delivery of human services, the problem of acceptance would be reason enough. An additional threat to locally organized and based services is the reluctance of trained professionals and of others in leadership positions to work in neighborhood settings — a serious long-term problem for these efforts.

For mental health services, all of these issues represent a peculiar closing of a circle. Responsibilities that were assumed by the state because they were handled so poorly by localities are now being returned to neighborhoods and local areas because they have been handled so poorly, in turn, by the state. At the core of the issue of decentralization is the problem of how services are to be linked in practice in the interest of problem solving for the patient or client. Experience would seem to indicate that because such linkages can occur only at the local level, they will therefore be achieved differently in different localities. This means, of course, that service systems will be diverse rather than uniform. Day-to-day management of programs should reside locally, not centrally, and each locale must make its own decisions as to how services will be integrated and how priorities will be set within overall state policy and funding. These local decisions will need to be made in a collaborative manner by those who provide services, those who utilize them, and those who pay for them.

Categorical Services in an Integrated Service System

Those interested in human services development have tended to mistake comprehensiveness as a planning concept for integrated services as a reality. Those who take this view fail to recognize that regardless of how it is accomplished, human services must be divided into manageable pieces. Certainly at state and national levels, the geography is too massive, the population too large, and, however comprehensive and integrated our thinking, the practical problems are simultaneously too numerous and too different for it to be otherwise.

Integrated services refers to the making of diverse service elements a whole, a unit, by bringing all the parts together — that is, to join the parts, to unite them. In contrast, categorical services are the technically specific elements or classes out of which the larger integrated system is constructed. Categorical services refer in this context to mental health services which exist in one system, social services which exist in another, medical services which exist in yet a third, and so forth. Another misapprehension exists that service categories are neither important nor germane to problems as people experience them. The development of specialized services had represented a step toward improved quality of both individual and institutional providers. It may be useful to keep in mind that whereas a systems analyst sees multiple problems, the client/patient may see a single (categorical) issue, and this is, after all, the client's choice.

A tendency also exists to equate categorical services with a categorical service system. According to this sort of thinking, educational services would be provided only in schools, health services only in hospitals and clinics, social services only in family service agencies. In fact, however, categorical services, and those specially trained to provide them (for example, physicians, social workers, and rehabilitation counselors), will be necessary in any service system no matter how comprehensively designed it may be. The problem is how to design a comprehensive and effective system that utilizes the skills of those who have been categorically trained in order to solve specific problems as they are experienced by the client.

Accessibility and Eligibility

A central theme of the human services concept has been the commitment to a one-tiered system offering services to all, rich and poor, as those services are required. According to this view, a determination of the need for service on the part of an individual or family must be divorced both from the ability to pay for the service and from its actual availability; only in this way will it be possible to estimate the size of the residual ("real") demand for service when not artificially limited by fiscal and other barriers. While the goal of making services readily available to all seems clear, the commitment of society to the sort of funding this would require is by no means clear.

Financing

Issues of cost and of methods for raising revenue for human service systems have become important matters of public concern. Since the demand for human services of various kinds appears to be unending for the forseeable future, there is no limit (defined by demand) on the sums that could be spent in this area.

Yet another mistaken belief which exists in this field is that integrating and bringing together various services for people will result in dramatic dollar savings. While conceivably true in the short-run, this has no long-term validity. Integrated delivery systems, utilizing rationalized management and administrative groupings organized on a geographic basis and incorporating specialized services will, in fact, save money in the short-run as movement away from less rationalized and less orderly groupings occurs. However, while it may be possible to reduce the unit cost of a service, it does not seem possible to reduce total expenditures without also reducing total services.

Manpower Utilization and Accountability

A further misconception to which the human services are subject is that those who work in these services, particularly in the public sector, are lazy, incompetent, cannot find a job elsewhere, and lack accountability. Given the frustration citizens often encounter when dealing with the various governmental bureaucracies, this view is understandable. But wide experience indicates that public-sector programs are, more often than not, staffed by hard-working, eager, and surprisingly flexible people who, if given the chance, will perform with competence and often in creative ways. However, public-sector employees, in particular, seldom are given the change. The complexities and rigidities of legislative, bureaucratic, and budget bureau control can stultify, suppress, indeed extinguish whatever initiative would otherwise be present.

With respect to public accountability, there is increasing acceptance that we must design systems in which service program managers are held accountable for the services they provide. Accountability is a complex issue which cannot be explored at length here [3,4]. Briefly stated, for those who provide services to be held accountable, there needs to be a situation of "risk" with the attendant possibility of success or failure. Given the low salaries for public service, the manager/worker at present runs the risk of failure without any possibility of potential reward for success. When politics and tax dollars are involved, the public is eager to expose failure and wary of claims of success.

Another kind of accountability regarding human service programs has received inadequate attention in the past but has recently become an area of increasing public attention. It focuses on the assessment and value of the content of the programs themselves instead simply of the adequacy with which they are managed. Appropriate questions are being addressed, insistently and persistently, to human service managers to justify in some quantitative (or even qualitative) fashion the expenditure of funds for which they are responsible. Evaluative studies in the human services field, even in that part of it pertaining to health services, have been few and in general inadequate [3]. As funding for social services programming becomes increasingly problemmatic, demands for evaluative information and program monitoring by those providing the funds will increase. If this results in a service system more tightly organized in terms of objectives, goals, and modalities, it may well prove a healthy step. Those involved in the social services, however, should not fall victim to the misconception that they will justify their services and their existence by "cost:benefit ratios" alone [3]. While management technology permits the comparison of one program option with another (to the degree these can be rationally quantified), it must not be allowed to trespass into the area of value judgments concerning the ways in which society chooses to allocate its resources.

A final word may be in order with respect to the utilization of new kinds of personnel. The human services movement has been built in part upon the earlier experience of the war on poverty programs which demonstrated that individuals of differing backgrounds could be trained to perform a wide range and variety of tasks and services in the health and social service sphere. One important new function has already emerged. Workers are required whose ongoing responsibility is to ensure that service agencies actually respond to client problems. This need exists because no system is conceivable under which all human services in a locality will be grouped with complete convenience to all and linked with total success, one to another. Instead of hoping for a perfect system, it is necessary to design one that takes account of the gaps remaining unclosed and provides a net (in this instance, specially trained staff) to recover those caught in the gaps. It is a mistake to believe, however, that the better allocation of tasks inherent in the use of new professionals and paraprofessionals will replace the specialized training of those in the previously existing professions. New workers may actually increase the unit cost of service (i.e., add to personnel costs without increasing volume or productivity) unless tasks and supervision are carefully redefined to free existing staff, and unless training is specific to need.

Service Delivery and Service Regulation

While not a necessary element of a human services approach, the concept of separating service from regulatory responsibilities has paralleled the evolution of human service organizations. The issue of whether to separate or link public provision of mental health services with provider and institutional licensing authority is an example. The pressure for improved quality of state-financed and delivered services has mitigated toward applying to those services the same standards increasingly being applied to services provided by the private sector. Indeed, this era is one in which public and private agencies are becoming increasingly indistinguishable; both depend overwhelmingly on public dollars for their support and both are increasingly being held to public account for the nature and quality of what they do.

A concurrent development has involved extension of the concept of regulation from the health field into the allied human services. Social and child care agencies, for example, are increasingly the object of state regulation regarding quality of care and allowable charges for services. This is a trend which will continue, in all likelihood, and is probably one component of the increasing irritation many citizens feel with government.

Prevention

Like deinstitutionalization, cost effectiveness and accessibility, prevention has become a shibboleth and an icon for those involved in "the human services." Some forms of prevention do work. There is no question that early intervention at the neighborhood level reduces the use of state hospitalization. There is also no question that patients who spend less time in state hospitals are less subject to developing an institutionalization syndrome. This does not mean they are less subject to recurrence of illness, however. Nor does any of this mean that modalities for preventing the onset of illness in the first instance are currently available. (Perhaps the closest the mental health field has come in the area of prevention has involved the use of lithium for the prevention of recurrent manic-depressive episodes — a dramatic development in neuropharmacology for which there has been no social equivalent.) In ways unfortunately similar to the community mental health and child guidance movements before it, the new human services thrust appears to promise a panacea for the social and psychological ills which plague us by simply trying harder and spending more.

The child guidance movement preceding World War II for example aimed at prevention of adolescent and adult disorders through work with problems as they developed in the young child. The movement lost some of its momentum with the discovery that this early treatment did not, in fact, prevent the emergence of disorders later in life.

The lesson of all of this seems clear. Having achieved so little, with particular reference to primary prevention, it would be best to claim little. The demand from human service advocates for increased funding of preventive programs seems ill advised when the benefits of such programs seem so elusive. This proscription should not be taken as an excuse on the part of those who would prefer not to improve certain social or environmental conditions such as housing, job opportunities, and worker satisfaction which undoubtedly contribute to a happier and more satisfying life and have value in and of themselves. Many serious physicial and mental illnesses cannot, however, be eliminated simply by improving social conditions.

Conclusions

The era of the 1960s saw the emergence and recognition of the consumer interest

in the provision of services [2]. At the program as well as the conceptual level
the division of society into providers and consumers became a reality, energized,
in part, by Office of Economic Opportunity programs. Many new services
have been designed which have accommodated to citizen advice or control.
Often, this citizen involvement focused on a view of the provider as enemy and
adversary, and while situations occur where this may be so, this notion of the
provider, in fact or fancy, is not inherent in, and is even contrary to, the intent
of the human services movement. Instead, a collaborative model bringing together
those who provide services, those who contribute to their support, and those who
receive services may be a more realistic framework if any genuine progress in
service integration and service delivery is to occur.

The development of neighborhood psychiatry has coincided in time with
the evolution of the human services movement. Both focus on local service
delivery systems and both look upon their mandates in broad rather than narrow
perspective. For neighborhood psychiatry, the human services movement represents at once an opportunity and a threat. It is an opportunity because neighborhood psychiatric practice is heavily dependent upon the nexus of service systems
within which it is embedded. It is a threat because the pressure toward amalga-
mation of services places neighborhood psychiatry in jeopardy of losing its
individuality and identity.

Concern regarding the loss of independent identity is a national phenomenon,
not simply a local one. Many citizen groups formed over the years around
specific (categorical) client groups previously ignored by society remain skeptical
of the human services effort. Each of these organizations has fought long and
hard for the gains it has made. Each is naturally resistant to submerging its interests and power, just as success may seem near, to a broader, less tangible human
services goal which seems distant, if attainable at all.

Mental health services, for example, achieved their present degree of funding
and governmental support with the help of special interest groups (mental health
and mental retardation associations) in part because they divorced themselves
from the existing health and social services. This separation encouraged public
visibility, specific capacity to lobby, and the development of both citizen and
professional political and technical expertise. The citizens and professionals who
fought this fight are reluctant to endanger what they have won over the years.

The human services movement has offered the opportunity to rethink the
ways people are served and the kinds of problems for which they need service.
The myths and misconceptions accompanying the development of the movement
encompass a number of serious problems and misunderstandings that threaten
its very existence. Of these, the most important may be the belief that there are
simple solutions for complex problems; that from simply amalgamating, for example, every specialist's technique there will come integrated, comprehensive, and
coordinated human services of high quality and reasonable cost. But complicated
problems have complex solutions — to the degree they have solutions at all. No

one, best way will fit each client, each problem, each provider, or each neighborhood. Frameworks must be flexible enough to allow options in service delivery and to permit wide variation in different localities and under special circumstances.

A desire prevails for human services to be all things to all people. This misapprehension manifests itself, for example, in the myriad tasks social workers for departments of welfare around the country have been asked to perform. They have been required to determine eligibility for financial and medical assistance, and to counsel, inspect, refer, place, and supervise. In trying to do so much, they have lost the confidence of the people whom they serve, of the taxpayers who must pay the bill, and of themselves. This unfortunate experience illustrates the importance of separating functional tasks when trying to solve difficult organizational problems. Categorization and specialization become both useful and desirable when placed in the context of a comprehensive and integrated system of service for people which focuses on problems and clusters the skills needed to work with those problems.

From the client's point of view, in addition to quality, what is desired is choice, flexibility, and responsiveness — options, not rigid channels; flexibility, not simply efficiency; and warmth, not resistance. These are largely attitudinal factors having to do with the way people are and the way they work, as much as with the product they deliver and the structure and framework within which they do it. For all of these reasons, the human services movement may prove to be more philosophy and process than system and product; and the human services umbrella agency, embodying the concept translated into structure, has yet to prove it represents a forward step of lasting value.

References

1. Caplan, R. and Caplan, G. *Psychiatry and the Community in Nineteenth-Century America.* New York: Basic Books, 1969.
2. Richmond, J.B. *Currents in American Medicine—A Developmental View of Medical Care and Education.* Cambridge: Harvard University Press, 1969.
3. Richmond, J.B. and Scherl, D.J. Research in the Delivery of Health Services. In: *The American Handbook of Psychiatry,* Vol. VI. Hamburg, D.A. and Brodie, H.K.H. (eds.). New York: Basic Books, 1975.
4. Scherl, D.J. "Outpatient Psychiatric Centers—Accountable To Whom?" In: *The Outpatient Patient.* Tulipian, A.B. and Cutting, A.M. (eds.). New York: Bruner Mazel 1972.

4

Neighborhood Approaches to Mental Health Services

Arthur J. Naparstek and *Chester D. Haskell*

Mental health professionals have earnestly sought to bring services into the community arena. A result of this effort is the community mental health movement which has had a profound impact on service delivery.[a] During the past decade, however, in spite of significant reforms and many important research efforts, providers and consumers have not been satisfied. Many still claim that services are delivered in a fragmented manner, that they are often offered in an inefficient, duplicative, and bureaucratically confusing fashion, that they lack accountability, and that service delivery systems do not provide for attention to prolonged needs or for comprehensive analysis of the patient's problems.

In part, such judgments stem from our lack of knowledge concerning how different groups of people solve problems and cope with crises. Further, service delivery systems are often developed without regard to the unique elements of community and neighborhood life.

The efficacy of a mental health system depends largely on recognizing the proper context for delivery. Although important work has been carried out with regard to linking service delivery to poor neighborhoods, the results have been disappointing. Despite the rhetoric supporting community involvement, mental health professionals have shown little real understanding of the dynamics of urban life.

During the past two decades human problems have been defined in the context of macrosocial and economic forces, resulting in the belief that poverty was the central issue and that innovations were needed to reform social institutions and provide opportunities for mobility for poor people, particularly for blacks. By the late 1960s, however, there was widespread disillusionment with the effectiveness of the approach. Under the guise of administrative reform, the first

The work reported in this chapter was supported by funds from the National Institute of Mental Health, Grant #1 R01 MH26531-01.

[a]This chapter will use the terms "neighborhood" and "community" interchangeably. Although there have been many studies and policy papers using the two terms as the field of focus, it is still possible to raise fundamental questions of definition: What is a neighborhood? What is a community? The literature on neighborhoods and communities contains a multiplicity of definitions, none of which appears to have universal acceptance. The concepts are defined from a host of different perspectives and ideological frames of reference, a result being that the definitions are often useful in a theoretical context, but difficult to operationalize in administrative or policy terms.

Nixon administration began to dismantle the service change initiatives taken during the early part of the decade, justified by the alleged inefficient administration and organization of "great society" programs.

The assumptions and beliefs underlying the service initiatives and theoretical systems of the sixties and early seventies were not directed toward the micro aspects of problem solving in a neighborhood context. Nor were these past efforts explicitly directed to the universal problems of inequality, social injustice, and exclusion. In the sixties these issues were given attention, but only within the context of poverty; in the seventies they are not even discussed.

Policy Analysis and Social Theory

A recurring theme in mental health has been the search for new models for the delivery of services. Rather, a new analysis is needed on the notion that a neighborhood approach cannot be cast only in its own policy and program terms. First and foremost, it requires involvement from all concerned sectors in a city. Second, if it is to be successful, it must be pluralistic to meet the diverse needs of different groups of people. Third, if one particular lesson can be learned from both the successes and failures of neighborhood level approaches, it is the need for "approachable scale." This is not a question of absolute size, but rather, what scale is appropriate for what we are trying to do. Small is not necessarily better than large, nor is neighborhood necessarily better than city. Some activities are best carried out at a larger scale than the neighborhood where the conventional notions of "economies of scale" come into play. In Schumacher's words, "for his different purposes, man needs many different structures, both small ones and large ones, some exclusive and some comprehensive" [1].

Money, or cost savings, is not and should not be the prime rationale for alterations in the ways in which services are delivered. The discomfort of America's urban populace is not solely related to quantifiable issues such as the cost of services or fee for service rates. Rather, a profound alienation pervades cities, encompassing feelings of powerlessness, meaninglessness, isolation, and self-estrangement. An underlying problem is thus, whether the roots of alienation can be found in the neighborhood, and whether human services can make a difference in reversing or negating those elements of community life which alienate.

Alienation and community are two central sociological concepts. However, each concept is extremely broad, laden with value implications, and has been used in an extraordinary variety of ways. Such social theorists as Toennies, Marx, Weber, Durkheim, and Simmel are perhaps most responsible for providing the "content" of the twentieth-century use of the word "alienation." Each conceptualized community in order to identify on a theoretical level the processes leading toward the depersonalization of human relations and intensification of the alienation process in community.

Although it is not the purpose of this chapter to discuss these theoretical constructs, if we are to reanalyze current programs it is important to identify central themes which flow through the work of these theorists. Two themes are dominant: one, when a person is unable to participate, control, or understand the processes shaping his social being, he will feel a sense of deprivation, dependency and manipulation; and two, alienating conditions arise when the community or the institutions in that community are unresponsive to the needs of the individual.

Thus, the failure of many community mental health efforts results from two interrelated problems: first, in most cases these efforts do not deal directly with the issues of devolving power to citizens on a neighborhood level; and second, the administrative arrangements of the formal mental health system are not supportive of a process consistently responsive to the needs of different groups of people. The remainder of this chapter will discuss the problem of devolving power in more specific terms and identify several options for linking services to neighborhoods.

Principles Guiding the Devolution of Power

Resource allocation must be a fundamental component of any strategy to devolve power. Policies which do not consider the ways in which citizens can control the allocation of resources are inadequate. No public or private agency exists in the country that does not in some way or other follow a strategy of resource allocation to neighborhoods. Monies and services are usually distributed to different neighborhood service districts on the basis of need as perceived by a small number of decision makers. Often the criteria for defining need is determined by a complex convergence of administrative, political, and economic forces, often having little to do with the true citizen needs of a particular neighborhood.

On the other hand, citizens determine their resource needs quite subjectively, utilizing criteria that are different from the professional. In assessing needs, citizens are guided by two interrelated principles: equity and sufficiency.

Equity

The principle of equity is defined by citizens in two ways: whether their investment (objective or subjective) is equal to their return; and whether their neighborhood is getting its fair share of resources as compared to other parts of the city. Thus, when citizens invest through the tax system, they expect a return in services and amenities. However, the problem is complicated in that the return is not within the complete control of the citizens or even local decision makers. Often, even well-intentioned policies developed on a national level can be extremely disruptive on a local level. An example of this is the impact of the Community Mental Health Centers Act of 1963. The Act was a part of the federal government's commitment to end poverty and racial discrimination. This legislation, together with the 1964 Economic Opportunity Act, could be considered a unique form of race and class legislation: it designated a special group in the population as eligible for the benefits of the law.

A working alliance between psychiatrists, social and political scientists, federal bureaucrats, and others attempted to forge a national effort that would serve local communities through mental health centers. But by 1970 these alliances broke down, and public support for the war on poverty and the CMHC Act dramatically abated.

The social policies of the 1960s drew lines: the policy makers in effect said, "Whites don't have problems—these people do." The anger and hostility felt by whites is not a result of their lack of sympathy for needs of the poor and blacks, but stems rather from a perception of inequity and a sense of being left out and ignored.

S. M. Miller contends that efforts to improve the circumstances of the poor will inevitably affect those groups economically and socially contiguous to them. Miller explained that in 1968 the group of people who had incomes between $3,450 (for a family of four—the 1968 poverty line) and approximately $10,000 ($9,750—income figure set by the United States Bureau of Labor Statistics as an "adequate but modest standard") felt ignored and neglected. He claimed that the responsibility for those feelings lay with the war on poverty and a sense that workers in this income range were "picking up the tab" for the poor.

Indeed, many feel that they are "put upon" by these efforts at change, bearing the burdens with little support and aid from the society at large. The likelihood is that these nonaffluent, but nonpoor groups will be calling for social services and other aids for themselves. Not only will they be seeking social services as mobility aids (for they too feel that their and their children's economic mobility is limited) but they will call for social services as basic amenities to which they have a claim [2].

Neither the great society programs nor the Community Mental Health Centers Act could have possibly fulfilled the expectations of their various constituencies. Rather than introducing the neighborhood programs through successive stages of accomplishment and functional expansion, the reverse occurred: a full dose of decentralization was introduced to an unorganized, and often overwhelmed, neighborhood populace. When neighborhood residents were unable to fulfill the mandate of these programs, the delivery system retrenched into greater centralization by reducing the devolution of control.

These programs tended to be defined in the context of race and an absolute definition of poverty. Thus, programs originally intended to serve the poor were quickly perceived (with even greater selectivity) as programs designed primarily for poor blacks. Though in most cities these categorical programs began on a small scale, they grew in time and attained a high visibility. The mandate of great society policies related to neighborhood control and service decentralization. Thus, neighborhood residents became actively involved and anxiously waited for their neighborhood conditions to improve. By 1968, subjective judgments evaluating the policies' impact in program terms were harsh. Tom Wicker comments that the war on poverty "somehow managed to wind up alienating many of the black and poor, as well as white conservatives . . . and members of Congress" [3]. Lee Rainwater notes that "though the E.O.A. [Economic Opportunity Act] made promises to the black community through its pseudo-radical rhetoric, it angered and insulted the working class, and at the same time delivered no more than symbolic resources to black people" [4].

Important lessons can be learned from these community-oriented policies. Robert Wood's analysis of the policies of the sixties links the past to the present and provides a framework for discussing current efforts. Wood notes that a critical policy issue raised in the sixties involved the complications inherent in the majority system working on a minority problem. He points out that policies which fail to take into account the economic and social needs of a majority are likely to stimulate fears which, in turn, override the minority needs:

The critical factor is how minority needs are presented to a majority and coupled with them, not the impossibility of gaining majority approval. This requires skill and leadership of special proportions [5].

Implicit in Wood's analysis are the skills needed to generate a process which will confront conditions of inequity as perceived by different groups of people.

We know that on a local level, actual or perceived states of inequity have significant consequences. For example:

1. if residents have sufficient resources they will opt out of the neighborhood and refuse to invest socially, physically, and economically;
2. or, residents will feel threatened by those they regard as below them in social and economic status, a consequence of which is increased hostility toward those who are considered to be different;
3. if a local agency projects an appearance of responsiveness, but does not fully permit power to be shared, people feel cheated and manipulated, resulting in an apartheid system of service delivery: minorities receive inadequate care, and poor and working class whites are caught in between—too poor to afford their own physicians but unwilling to attend a public-supported center.

Sufficiency

This principle is defined in terms of people being able to participate in processes of service delivery and to exercise some degree of control over these services so they have the ability to deal successfully with the problems confronting their community. When these conditions do not exist, one can expect levels of alienation which, in turn, negatively influence the self-perceptions of one's neighborhood.

The degree to which people feel sufficient is often determined by how the neighborhood defines itself and how others define it. Neighborhoods which have strong ethnic, racial, or class identities often tend to have the greatest ability to deal with their problems. Such neighborhoods have a unique sense of pride which, in turn, affects the ways in which they resolve difficulties. Yet public officials and scholars often refer to these communities in condescending, often perjorative terms, policy makers do not build on the strengths of the neighborhood and do not understand neighborhood social and cultural dynamics.

In order to discuss the linkages between service delivery systems and neighborhoods, the infrastructure of the neighborhood—that is, those neighborhood-based networks (organizational and cultural) which can increase accountability between the "system" and the citizens—is of critical importance. When such networks do not operate effectively, a low level of citizen involvement can be expected in areas of service delivery and a high level of mistrust between consumers and providers.

Although important work has been carried out with regard to linking service delivery to neighborhoods, little consideration has been given to neighborhoods with multiethnic populations. We have not developed a full understanding of the intercultural dimensions of neighborhood life, particularly as it relates to service delivery. Too often delivery systems bypass those neighborhood-based cultural and organizational networks which may have the potential for support of services. More specifically, the impact of different ethnic groups and subcultures on issues related to prevention and treatment is not fully understood. Finally, the problem is made more complex because we do not yet know empirically what the possibilities and ramifications of the interdependencies of race, ethnicity, social class, and well being are for neighborhood service delivery.

Ethnicity, Social Class and Well Being

Human service delivery systems are usually organized according to the perceptions of "what is needed" by the providers, who, for the most part neither live in the neighborhoods where the service centers are located, nor reflect the same socioeconomic or cultural background as their "consumers." An important difference between professional and client perceptions of need thus exists. And this difference mitigates against developing the sensitivity necessary for understanding not only the relationship of utilization patterns of human services to social, religious and ethnic factors, but also in what ways and to what degree they are linked.

The relationship between well being and ethnicity builds on the work of Mead, Benedict, and Kluckhohn, as well as Sullivan, Horney, Ferenczi, and Kardiner—all of whom stressed the influence of social and cultural environment on normal and deviant behavior. The work of Kolodny [6], Spiegal [7], Barrabe and Von Mering [8], and Zborowski [9] suggest that various ethnic groups differ in their responses to health, illness, and treatment. However, there is a lack of empirical evidence which links utilization patterns to ethnic variation [10].

Only recently have some of the interrelationships between social class and mental health been specified. The classic work of Hollingshead and Redlich bridged the gap between mental health and social class by raising two fundamental questions: (1) Is mental health or illness related to social class? (2) Does a patient's position in the status system affect the treatment she or he receives? [11] One conclusion drawn from this study was that occupation is a potent force in determining a person's general life adjustments and ways of coping with problems. This conclusion is also supported by Srole's Midtown Manhattan Study [12] and the Gurin, Veroff, and Field nationwide survey of 2,400 adults [13]. Further, the work of Gurin and Strole, together with that of Leighton [14] and Phillips [15] has shown that as many as 50 percent of those who have emotional problems never seek and receive any kind of help.

Finally, these investigations demonstrate that the world of semi-skilled and unskilled blue collar workers produces a life situation of deprivation, insecurity, and powerlessness resulting in fear, frustration, and a sense of helplessness and low self-esteem. The work of Kornhauser [16], Mills [17], and Fromm [18] support the aforementioned conclusion and strongly imply the work people do has important consequences for their ego strengths.

In summary, this literature provides some empirical evidence indicating that various ethnic groups differ in their responses to health, illness, and treatment and that by utilizing occupation as a principal indicator of social class we move closer to establishing a causal relationship between work and behavior. However, the relationships between ethnic variation, occupation, and utilization rates are not clear. For example, can it be assumed that a large majority of workers identify themselves as "ethnic"? If so, does ethnicity or occupation have the more powerful impact on prevention and treatment? Giordano's review of the literature [19] responds to the latter question and suggests that ethnicity has at least as powerful an impact on mental health and mental illness as social class. He points out that the influence of ethnicity becomes particularly significant in those studies where social class is held constant. However, he notes that while professionals have already accepted class differentials, ethnic

variation is still often ignored, or worse, denied outright. Thus, ethnicity and
sufficiency would appear to be closely related.

Neighborhood-Based Cultural and Organizational Networks

Another body of literature shows the importance of neighborhood-based networks, providing clues as to how people solve their problems and cope with
crises when they are outside the system of professional agencies. In their study
of social class and mental illness, Myers and Bean [20] point out that for those
in the professional system, the effectiveness of help received will depend on the
social supports or lack of support in a person's neighborhood. The importance
of neighborhood-based cultural or organizational networks for assisting professionals deal with the physically and mentally ill has been noted by such scholars
as Slater [21], Glazer [22], Warren [23], Litwak [24], and Breton [25]. For
example, Glazer notes that a significant contribution to the present crisis in public social policy and service delivery is due to the breakdown of "traditional"
organizations and ways of dealing with problems. Breton, analyzing the issue
from the ethnic dimension, points out that greater attention should be given to
the social organizations (fraternal organization, ethnic clubs, and so forth) of
ethnic communities and particularly to the wide variation among them.

By avoiding existing neighborhood-based networks we make it more difficult for people to utilize professional expertise in effective and differentiated
ways. Therefore, important questions arise as to how people who are not a
part of neighborhood service delivery systems cope with their problems. What
neighborhood-based formal and informal networks of service delivery are being
used? What rearrangements of the formal delivery systems are necessary so that
the social organization within the neighborhood is strengthened? Will a delivery
system which is culturally compatible with the neighborhood increase utilization and reach people earlier in their illness?

Policy Implications for the Future

Although the CMHC program has survived the dismantling of the Economic
Opportunity Act, its future is still cloudy. David Musto points out that the
future of the mental health service delivery system will be determined by the
form of national health insurance that emerges in the next few years [26].
In any event, service delivery in a neighborhood context is a prevalent and recurring issue today. Often it is cast in terms of breaking up a centralized service delivery system and moving toward decentralization. This concept has
arisen in response to a number of overlapping and ill-defined pressures and
forces, a major example being the sharp rise in demand for human services.

Kahn and others have pointed to this phenomenon, locating some of its origins in the multiethnic characters of our larger cities: postwar emigration that resulted in the juxtaposition of numerous ethnic groups in relatively narrow physical spaces, with each having its own needs and methods of coping with crises [27]. A companion factor has been the differing, problematic, and complex ways in which diverse classes and age groups are affected by the realities of modern urban life.

An additional force toward decentralization is the recognition by the public officials that real inequities exist in the distribution of public services and resources among the city's neighborhoods. The result is a competitive climate in which alienation is further encouraged when the residents of one neighborhood feel that their community is getting less than a "fair deal" relative to others. They articulate the problem in terms of political clout—and, of course, the perception of its absence does little to enhance their faith in "downtown" capability, concern, or responsiveness.

Finally, the tendency toward decentralization has received impetus from the federal sector in the form of funding. The CMHC Act and Great Society programs, with their common emphasis on citizen involvement, set the foundation for legitimate client involvement in the program process. In addition to providing a strong impetus for such participation, these mandates legitimized citizen activity and even created a revolution of rising expectations among those citizens who believed they really should be involved in the processes by which their lives are affected.

The experience of the sixties suggests that decentralization of services and a straight resource approach to neighborhoods in isolation will not support a viable neighborhood climate. Although the community mental health movement was predicated on the notion that its programs could improve the overall quality of community life, little attention has been given by mental health professionals to the complex set of legal, administrative, and fiscal policies which independently and/or collectively make it difficult or impossible to bring about change. These obstacles to change are often structural aspects of the urban system and create a set of negative incentives for neighborhood viability. For example, neighborhoods cannot maintain a viable infrastructure (network) if local and state policies, ordinances, regulations, and judicial decisions affect a community negatively. Further, such public actions often serve as legal obstacles which inhibit participation and foster a sense of insufficiency among residents. Another example of a negative incentive is the relationship between general municipal services and neighborhood approaches to the human services. Interdependence among the differing components involved in the delivery of various types of service is essential to a healthy community environment. Inequitable distribution of city services stimulates conditions in which people will not stay in a given neighborhood, serving to erode neighborhood-based networks and thus permit and engender conditions of inequity and insufficiency. Thus, a primary precondition for change must be the identification of such negative incentives, their removal, and the concomitant creation of incentives for the maintenance and enhancement of neighborhood-based networks.

The decisions facing local mental health professionals on neighborhood-related issues are complex and politically hazardous. Often practitioners are confronted with a dwindling tax base, aging housing stock, increased numbers of aged and dependent people, underemployment, and a breakdown in public service delivery systems. These problems, in turn, lead to varied conditions of alienation and make it difficult to decentralize services in any meaningful way. Further, these conditions foster the practice of triage: having to choose between services to white middle-class families who are threatening to leave the city, and services to the poor and minorities.

Current thought now focuses on the integration of mental health and health policies and programs. However, there is a prior issue: development of policies on local, state, and federal levels which can support the viability of neighborhoods. Only within the context of a comprehensive neighborhood policy can we hope for the successful implementation of a community mental health strategy. For only if neighborhoods are strong can they serve as the proper context for service delivery.

Enactment of an Omnibus Neighborhood Act is needed in order to facilitate a comprehensive approach toward restructuring the processes of governance through a mix of centralization and decentralization of public and human services. Further, legislation aimed at eliminating systemic origins of neighborhood decline and restructuring financial systems with an emphasis on linking subsidy and incentive programs to neighborhood-based networks need to be developed. Perhaps the greatest challenge of all confronting community psychiatry and the human services is the linking of federal funds and programs to local conditions and strengths in ways which will increase utilization and decrease racial tension and polarization.

References

1. Schumacher, E. F., *Small is Beautiful: Economics as if People Mattered* (New York: Perennial) 1973.
2. Mill, S. M. and Altschuler, J., "Services for People," Report of the Task Force on Organization of Social Services (U.S. Department of Health, Education, and Welfare) February, 1968.
3. *The New York Times*, July 28, 1968.
4. Rainwater, L., "Making the Good Life: Working Class Family and Life Style" (unpublished manuscript) October, 1970.

5. Wood, R., *The Necessary Majority: Middle America and the Urban Crisis* (New York: Columbia University Press) 1972.

6. Kolodny, R., "Ethnic Cleavages in the United States," *Social Work*, XIV, January, 1969.

7. Spiegel, J., "Some Cultural Aspects of Transference and Counter Transference," in Zold, M. W. ed. *Social Welfare Institutions* (New York: Wiley & Sons), 1965.

8. Barrabe, P. and Von Mering, O., "Ethnic Variation in Mental Stress in Families with Psychotic Children," *Social Problems*, I, October, 1953.

9. Zborowski, *People in Pain* (San Francisco: Joseey-Bass) 1964.

10. Annotated Bibliography on Ethnicity and Ethnic Groups, Kolm, R., ed., (Rockville, MD, NIMH) 1973.

11. Hollingshead, A. and Redlich, F., *Social Class and Mental Illness* (New York: Wiley & Sons, 1958).

12. Srole, L., Lagner, T., Michael, S., Opler, M. and Rennie, T., *Mental Health in the Metropolis: The Midtown Manhattan Study* (New York: McGraw Hill) 1962.

13. Gurin, G., Veroff, J., and Field, S., *Americans View Their Mental Health* (New York: Basic Books) 1960.

14. Leighton, A., *My Name is Legion.* (New York: Basic Books) 1959.

15. Phillips, D., "The True Prevalence of Mental Illness in a New England State," *Community Mental Health Journal* 2:1, Spring, 1966.

16. Kornhauser, A., "The Mental Health of Factory Workers: A Detroit Study," *Human Organization,* Vol. 21, 1962.

17. Mill, C. Wright, *White Collar: The American Middle Classes* (New York: Oxford University Press, 1951); *The Power Elite* (New York: Oxford University Press, 1959).

18. Fromm, E., *The Sane Society* (New York: Holt, Rinehart and Winston) 1955.

19. Giordano, J., *Ethnicity and Mental Health.* (New York: American Jewish Committee) 1973.

20. Myers, J., and Bean, L., A Decade Later: *A Follow-Up of Social Class and Mental Illness* (New York: Wiley & Sons) 1968.

21. Slater, P., *The Pursuit of Loneliness: American Culture at the Breaking Point* (Boston: Beacon Press) 1970.

22. Glazer, N., "The Limits of Social Policy" *Commentary*, 52:3, September, 1971.

23. Warren, D., "Neighborhood in Urban Areas," *The Encyclopedia of Social Work* (New York: NASW) 1971.

24. Litwak, E., "Voluntary Associations and Neighborhood Cohesion," *American Sociological Review*, 26:2, April, 1961.

25. Breton, R., "Institutional Completeness of Ethnic Communities and the Personal Relations of Immigrants," *American Journal of Sociology*, Vol. 70, 1964. pp. 193-205.

26. Musto, D., "Whatever Happened to Community Mental Health," *The Public Interest*, No. 39, Spring, 1975.

27. Kahn, A., "Service Delivery at the Neighborhood Level: Experience, Theory, and Fads," presented at the Symposium on Neighborhood Service Delivery, Community Service Society of New York, October, 1974.

5

Perspectives on Neighborhood Health Centers

Diana Chapman Walsh and
William J. Bicknell

More a concept than a coherent entity, neighborhood health centers are "many things to many people." A review of some perspectives on their development and operation provides additional dimensions for understanding their function as an important context for neighborhood psychiatry.

With historical roots reaching at least as far back as the early 1900s [1] they embodied in the 1960s a recognition on the part of federal strategists in the war on poverty that health, very broadly defined, would necessarily constitute a major battlefront [2]. Supported originally through research and demonstration funds from the Community Action Program in the Office of Economic Opportunity (OEO), they rapidly outgrew their status as demonstration projects and became, over time, "the most extensive concerted public effort in the history of the United States to expand ambulatory health care resources in poverty communities on a nationwide basis."[3]   In their heyday, neighborhood health centers developed in two directions: they were part of a broad social movement [4] seeking to intervene at the community level in the "cycle of poverty", and they evolved into a health movement with an identity and constituency all their own.

Today neighborhood health centers symbolize at once two contradictory realities: on the one hand, a nearly complete retrenchment from the war on poverty and the idealistic values it expressed, and on the other, continuing efforts to restructure the health care delivery system. Efforts in the latter direction focus on improving equity of distribution and access to care, and moving the center of the system away from its emphasis on urban and suburban hospital-based, episodic, specialty medicine toward comprehensive and continuous primary care for all, attuned to the psychosocial and environmental dimensions of health.

Neighborhood health centers were and are a varied collection of delivery vehicles, characterized by a diversity which confounds generalization, which may be the fountainhead of their strength. For if one were forced to single out the most critical factors in the development of neighborhood health centers, those would be the breadth and sweep of the objectives set for them, the latitude they were given, the flexibility allowed, and the requirement that they be tailored to the specifications and convenience not of the providers but of the consumers. All of these, in turn, foreordained their diversity.

Impetus and Evolution

In the wave of antipoverty legislation initiated in the early 1960s, neighborhood health centers found support from several sources—OEO and other federal programs, notably Title V of the Social Security Act (Maternal and Infant Care, Children and Youth Projects), administered by the Department of Health, Education and Welfare, and the Model Cities Program, administered by the Department of Housing and Urban Development, as well as from local health departments and small private foundations.

But the prototypes were the neighborhood health centers funded first by OEO, later by HEW, through section 314(e) of the 1967 Partnership for Health Act. Beginning in the summer of 1965, the original three grants were made by OEO's Community Action Program (CAP); five more projects were approved for funding by midway through the following summer. In November, 1966, an amendment to the Economic Opportunity Act, introduced by Senator Edward M. Kennedy, established the OEO Comprehensive Health Service Program and earmarked funds to develop neighborhood health centers in order to:

assure that [health] services are made readily accessible to residents of . . . areas [of concentrated poverty], are furnished in a manner most responsive to their needs and with their participation, and, whenever possible, are combined with . . . arrangements for providing employment, education, social or other assistance needed by the families and individuals served [5].

The Kennedy Amendment obviated an important controversy. Those in the federal government who had felt that OEO's efforts in health should be designed to close particular gaps in the services available in a given community had been outflanked by advocates of a more radical approach: comprehensive care was to be emphasized and programs undertaken "that could have significant influence in changing the health care delivery system." [6]

A $51 million Congressional appropriation followed in 1967, and with it the approval of another 33 neighborhood health center projects [2]. Congress reduced the allocation to $33 million the next year, but the program continued to expand in size [6]. By 1971, OEO grants had established about 100 neighborhood health centers; HEW funds made possible another 50 projects [3]. Approximately 104 of these projects were still in existence as of 1974, and were serving an estimated 1.3 million people [7]; see Table 5-1. Through 1971, the total federal investment in neighborhood health centers had exceeded $440 million, with individual grants normally falling within the $1 to 4 million range, and with projects located in roughly 120 different communities in 42 states [3].

Although the program continued to focus predominantly on the classic neighborhood health center model, other strategies for improving the primary care available to the poor were also tried. After the first two rounds of funding,

Table 5-1

Neighborhood Health Center Registrants and Federal Project Grants, Fiscal Years, 1968-74

Fiscal Year	Number of Projects	Registrants (in thousands)		Federal Project Grants	
		Per Project	Total	Per Registrant	Total (in millions)
1968	51	2.6	135	$275	$ 37.1
1969	67	4.6	305	203	62.0
1970	89	6.5	576	174	100.0
1971	112	8.7	975	169	165.0
1972	110	11.6	1,281	139	174.9
1973	106	12.0	1,270	131	166.9
1974 (est).	104	13.5	1,400	141	198.0

Source: Reyholds, R.A. "Improving access to health care among the poor – the neighborhood health center experience," *Milbank Memorial Fund Quarterly/Health and Society* 54 (1):51, 1976. Reprinted with permission.

the original concept of a neighborhood health center serving communities of from 20,000 to 30,000 saw expansions and modifications. Efforts were made beginning in 1970 to restructure outpatient departments of hospitals so that they might provide comprehensive primary care to neighboring low income communities. In effect, the hospitals were being encouraged to organize themselves to perform effectively a role they had long filled haphazardly and by default. In addition, community health network programs were developed in hopes of serving larger populations (of about 100,000), using a prepaid model with a sliding fee scale to encourage service to a more heterogeneous population including, under one roof, the poor, the near-poor, and the nonpoor, and coordinating a wide variety of existing health and social services. None of these more ambitious projects, however, came as close to achieving its full potential as did the freestanding neighborhood health center, largely because, as a group, they did not receive the broad social support and intense technical assistance from the federal government which was an integral part of the initial OEO approach.

Underlying Principles

Global, idealistic, and in the end, neither fully attainable nor even readily or effectively measurable, the goals and principles originally envisaged for neighborhood health centers were nonetheless well in line with the problems they sought to confront [3]. Just as health care was drawn into the war on poverty in response to the reality that equality of economic opportunity was often precluded by physical impairments and ill health [2], so too did the reverse appear true. No amount of medical care *per se*, however well organized and rendered, would materially improve the lot of people living in dire poverty, whose housing was unfit for human habitation, whose water supply was contaminated, or who were malnourished and perennially hungry [8]. Health, then, would have to be defined in very broad terms.

This was a fundamental principle, and it justified numerous experiments addressing community, environmental, and occupational health issues, as well as innovations ranging even farther afield—legal, agricultural, economic—all aimed ultimately at breaking the poverty cycle. The patient was to be viewed in his family and community context, and the services available to him, including mental health, were to be coordinated and integrated. OEO deliberately wrote very general guidelines intended to stimulate innovation, and at times found that they were being taken too literally, construed too narrowly by people in the field uncomfortable with the ambiguity of not knowing precisely what the funding source wanted.

Of particular relevance to the field of neighborhood psychiatry, the broad definition of health emanated in large part from a strong orientation among those involved in the early design of neighborhood health centers toward community mental health. Many of the physicians in Washington involved in developing the program were psychiatrists who came to perceive the centers not as medical care programs with a mental health component, but rather, in their totality, as strategies for community mental health intervention or vehicles for involving large numbers of community members in activities aimed at primary prevention of mental illness [9]. This perception was subtle and seldom overtly articulated; it was certainly not in the thinking of the neighborhood people actually developing centers. But it is an important part of the philosophical and theoretical heritage of neighborhood health centers.

The second major principle—maximum community participation—related closely to the first, was, in fact, almost a corollary. The populations to be served were to be intensely involved in the health centers, both as parties to decision making and as paid employees. However halting the early implementation of this principle may have been, from the outset the OEO "healthrights" program took seriously the Community Action Program commitment to community participation.

Consumer participation was thus viewed as both an end in itself and a means to the third broad principle: that services be convenient and acceptable to their potential users and that they be provided with dignity and continuity. The two levels of participation of community members—as board members in the formulation of policy and as trained staff members in the delivery of services—were designed theoretically to bridge the gap between the providers and the low-income community. In practice, the theory was not without its weaknesses [8], particularly during the early years before issues of power and control began to be resolved.

Distinctive Characteristics

The principal ingredients of neighborhood health centers evolved over time and were, to a large extent, evoked by the succession of individual applications for project grants. Although generalization is hazardous, the basic characteristics of neighborhood health centers are usually evident in four broad categories: (1) organizational structure, (2) physical location and target population, (3) type and scope of services, and (4) staffing patterns.

Organizational Structure

From the outset, grants deliberately bypassed state and most local institutional structures, flowing directly from the Executive Office of the President to the corporate entity administering the center. In the early years, this entity was most often a local health care institution (a hospital, medical school, or health department) which was then charged with organizing a consumer advisory board [3], usually comprising equal numbers of providers, community leaders, and consumers. As a result, the original enthusiasm for the program came more from providers than from consumers [2], and early organizational structures tended to give the control to existing health care institutions. Token community participation shifted gradually in many cases to actual consumer control, a shift that was invariably fraught with conflict [8].

Later years saw the flowering of single-purpose health corporations (Table 5-2), structures created for the express purpose of receiving the grant and administering the center, generally with consumers clearly and directly in control. The result proved a neater arrangement; with the underlying issue of control resolved, routine business could be conducted efficiently and problems addressed quickly. A responsiveness was possible with the single-purpose health corporation that was seldom achieved in the earlier, more cumbersome organizational framework.

Most centers have some degree of hospital affiliation, often with a teaching hospital. By 1972, over half the nation's teaching hospitals had been involved in some way in the development of neighborhood health centers [3].

Physical Location and Service Population

By definition, neighborhood health centers are located in the neighborhoods

Table 5-2
Administering Agencies of Projects Aided by OEO at Time of Initial Grant Award

Administering Agency	1965-6 %	1967 %	1968 %	1969 %	1970 %	1971 %
New health corporation		24	33	33	52	59
Hospital	50	21	22	67	9	10
Medical school	37	18	11		18	7
Health department	13	18	11			
Group practice		7			9	3
Other		10	22		13	21

Source: Zwick, D.I. "Some accomplishments and findings of neighborhood health centers," *Milbank Memorial Fund Quarterly/Health and Society* 50 (4):399, 1972. Reprinted with permission.

Note: In some cases the administering agency of a project has changed during the life of the project, usually from a medical school to a new health corporation.

they serve, and the initial intent was that those neighborhoods have high concentrations of poverty. In reality, the communities in which centers are situated vary widely as to the degree of poverty they contain [7]. Centers are located throughout the United States, "from northern Maine to the southern border of California to the western coast of Alaska." [3] About three fourths are in urban neighborhoods, the remainder in rural communities, in both instances less often heterogeneous ethnically than distinctly black, Chicano, or white.

A critical principle at the outset was that entitlement to services would not be based on income; residence alone would define a person's eligibility. This was dropped in 1967 when Congress passed an amendment stipulating that only poor people were eligible for the free services of neighborhood health centers; guidelines issued in 1968 specified standards of "closely related programs" (i.e., other OEO programs and Medicaid) [3]. Nonpoverty patients of neighborhood health centers are now required to pay for services, either directly out of pocket or through third-party coverage. The near-poor pay according to a sliding scale fee schedule. Nevertheless, a 1976 survey of registrants in 82 centers found that almost 90 percent are among the poor or near-poor [7]. Largely because centers have not developed exclusively in pockets of extreme poverty, they by and large have not become the community-wide resource of the early OEO vision [7].

Type and Scope of Services

Neighborhood health centers have striven "to organize and provide comprehensive ambulatory health care to individuals and families."[3] Centers are normally not divided into specialty clinics, and insofar as possible, a family is enrolled as a single unit. The basic service package comprises medical and dental care, laboratory and X-ray services, and usually on-site pharmacies. Most centers also administer home health and mental health programs, and provide social and community services and transportation. Supplemental services offered by some centers and not by others include such programs as physical or speech therapy, screening and treatment for sickle cell anemia or lead paint poisoning, optometry, or family planning [7] . Table 5-3 shows the distribution of these services in the 82 centers studied in 1976. Of particular interest here is the fact that 76% of the 82 neighborhood health centers studied provide direct mental health services and 94% provide social and community services. Efforts to reach out to the community in order to overcome non financial barriers to access are fundamental to neighborhood health centers. Some kind of out-reach program, usually staffed at least in part by trained community members as "family health workers" [10] or some variant thereof, has always been a key feature.

Table 5-3
Range of Services at 82 Neighborhood Health Centers

Service	% of Centers Offering Service
Direct health activities	
Mental health	76
Home health	83
Physical or speech therapy	26
Optometry	37
Sickle cell	40
Lead poisoning	31
Family planning	26
Supporting health activities	
Social and community services	94
Transportation	93
Training	81
Community organization	53
Environmental	67
Research and evaluation	29

Source: Reynolds, R.A. "Improving Access to Health Care Among the Poor – The Neighborhood Health Center Experience." *The Milbank Memorial Fund Quarterly/Health and Society* 54:61, 1976. Reprinted with permission.

Staffing

The neighborhood health center program has been an important focus and testing ground for "the team approach to primary health care."[11] In principle, the concept brings together primary physicians, mid-level practitioners, and family health workers in mutually supporting and intersecting roles designed to coordinate the medical and social services needed by each patient and his or her family. Instead of being the sole or principal provider of care, the physician becomes a supervisor and consultant, within his or her areas of expertise. The mid-level practitioner carries broad responsibility and frequently functions as leader of the team. Originally filled most often by a public health nurse or social worker, this role has, in recent years, come to be filled typically by a nurse practitioner or physician assistant.

Ideally, in concert with the physician, other team members broaden the scope of the care provided, increase the depth and subtlety of the understanding of each patient, and provide the means of placing medical and psychosocial needs within the broader context of family and community. In reality the ideal is elusive [12]. Physicians as currently trained are loathe to delegate responsibility and are inexperienced as supervisors [13]. Selection and training of all team members is crucial but is difficult and time consuming [11]. Moreover the rapid turnover rate of physicians practicing in neighborhood health centers [7] is hardly conducive to the slow, thoughtful process necessary to build effective primary care teams.

Problems and Promise: Lessons for the Future

It should come as no surprise that neighborhood health centers have, over the years, encountered myriad problems, large and small, and have surmounted some while simply side-stepping others. Difficulties and conflict were inevitable from the start, with so much at stake and the air so profoundly roiled. The program set out, in a single stroke, to redesign and alter the totality of primary care services for the poor—their physical location, organizational structure, mix of services, and staffing patterns.

The issue of how fairly to evaluate an effort so diffuse and broad in scope has never been fully resolved and many knotty problems remain. The question of how to weigh the value of the services rendered against some measure of unit cost, relative to traditional services which are more limited and not truly comparable has yet to be answered [3]. With services right in the community and with residents directly involved, confidentiality has been difficult to protect [14]. Political problems frequently go unresolved; conflict has often been vituperative and needlessly destructive [15]. Despite rhetoric to the contrary, services remain fragmented and integration at the neighborhood level has proven difficult and costly [16]. Team care and the physician assistant/nurse practitioner movement show promise, but much of it still unfulfilled [13]. Staffing in general has been complex and instability the rule: fewer than half of neighborhood health center physicians have remained in their jobs for more than two years, perhaps in part because the program as a whole has failed to gain adequate recognition from organized medicine [7]. Further, the danger has always existed that neighborhood health centers will isolate and segregate the poor, leaving them without choice as to where they will go for care [17], and creating what amounts to a separate (and potentially inferior) system of primary care for those unable to pay. One of the major failings has been that the strategy was developed for the poor and has not been generalized much beyond.

These problems ebb and flow, but the one issue overshadowing all others is the problem of long-term financing. OEO originally hoped to set in motion the neighborhood health center program, by providing front-end funding, then gradually to withdraw as centers developed the capacity to recoup operating expenses from Medicaid, and to a lesser extent from Medicare and other financing mechanisms. According to early projections, from 70 to 80 percent of health center costs would ultimately be reimbursable through Titles XVIII and XIX of the Society Security Act, both enacted in 1965, within a year of the launching of the neighborhood health center program. In time, however, it became painfully clear that these projections rested on a serious overestimate of the Medicaid program's promise. In reality only about 13 percent of neighborhood health center funds come from reimbursements (87 percent still come from project grants), and a 1973 Congressional study projected that at best about 20 percent of neighborhood health center costs could ever be expected to derive from Medicaid funds [7].

Buffeted by the manipulations and vagaries of state level politics, most state Medicaid programs are too limited—in eligibility ceilings, and/or scope of services covered—to be of much relevance to a service package aiming above all for comprehensiveness and continuity. Medicare, for the elderly, covers only a minor proportion of the clients of neighborhood health centers, and general escalation of the costs of providing health care has further exacerbated the problem of recouping operating expenses.

Contrary to original design, neighborhood health centers, for the most part, have failed to capture and combine the fragments of categorical health funds available to a given community. Although very comprehensive themselves, the centers have seldom been able to convince other programs drawing federal funds—maternal and child health, family planning, public health nursing—to pool resources with those of the neighborhood health center, to integrate services, and ultimately to build a single (and therefore larger and more powerful) resource for health care in the community. More recently there have been some successful attempts to involve CMHC's in providing some of the mental health services within neighborhood health centers.

Problems and shortcomings aside, neighborhood health centers have proved important points, have developed valuable models, have initiated some lasting change, and perhaps most importantly, have provided badly needed service, as well as a vehicle for learning and personal growth for providers and consumers alike.

It was demonstrated early and persistently [7,19] that neighborhood health centers were potentially acceptable, accessible and relevant to the needs of a population previously deprived of medical care. A 1976 evaluation [7] cites this as the most important policy question, and goes on to demonstrate that the centers "have been notably successful in removing barriers to health care among the poor." Assessments of the quality of the care rendered at neighborhood health centers have found it equal, sometimes superior, to the care available from other primary care providers [7,20].

The costs of neighborhood health centers, despite their broader services and different organizational structures, are competitive with those of other institutional providers, such as outpatient departments and clinics of hospitals and large prepaid group practices [16]. Economies of scale have been found to obtain: the cost per medical encounter ranges from $28.76 for centers with fewer than 5,000 registrants to $21.81 for those with 20,000 and more [7].

In line with their global objectives, neighborhood health centers have made varied and significant contributions beyond the realm of health care. They have served as a focus for constructive neighborhood action, out of which it has been possible to address a broad range of problems. They have offered employment and fostered economic development in the neighborhoods in which they are situated, highlighting the role of the health sector as an employer and an economic force in the community [21]. They have promoted a dialogue between the medical establishment and low income communities, have brought people together to learn about each other and have served as a mechanism for the airing and resolution of conflict. They have served as laboratory and classroom for low income people—teaching coping and organizing skills, giving entrée to the outside world, providing community people with staff and funds and allowing them to experiment with managing resources on their own behalf. The result in some communities has been the improvement of the image of the black male [22], in others it has stimulated solidarity among Chicano farm workers [22], in many it has contributed to a process of "growing taller."[3]

Neighborhood health centers have foreshadowed and sometimes paved the way for abiding changes in the planning, organization, and delivery of primary care services. The OEO model of consumer participation has fundamentally altered the rules governing planning and decision making in the health sector. Neighborhood health centers were at the forefront of the health consumers' movement, confronting hospitals and medical schools, challenging the right of the professionals to reserve for themselves all the power and influence. It seems unlikely that major decisions concerning the allocation of resources for health care will ever again be made through gentlemen's agreements reached behind closed doors [23].

The primary care movement, still gaining momentum, was itself an outgrowth of the neighborhood health center program, and so too the growing emphasis on team medicine and the full use of nonphysician manpower. This has also been the case with the newer developments in community mental health which this volume addresses. The cry for the development of alternatives to institutions—particularly alternatives to nursing homes and now state mental hospitals and perhaps also state schools for the mentally retarded—echoes important elements of the neighborhood health center strategy. Increasingly, it is recognized that some mechanism is needed, in the face of a fragmented and bewildering array of health and support services for the elderly and chronically disabled, to help these population groups negotiate the system or to do it on their behalf, and thus enable them to remain in their own homes and communities with independence and dignity intact. A neighborhood health center can be just such a mechanism, as evidenced by the pioneering home care programs for the elderly being developed within the neighborhood health center framework [24].

With financing issues not fully resolved, it still seems possible that neighborhood health centers will demonstrate their ability, as a local mechanism responsive to community needs, to take an ever changing resource mix and fashion out of it a program that makes sense for the people it serves. The longrange solution to the financial problems besetting neighborhood health centers may lie in national financing mechanisms and prepaid benefit packages [16]. An added advantage of this approach is the possibility that it would restore to low-income consumers the freedom to choose the locus of their care and would theoretically set up competition among alternative organizational structures and service packages vying for the primary care dollar.

Whatever may become of the concept, neighborhood health centers have focused a national spotlight on primary care and have taken important strides toward conceptualizing a form of comprehensive ambulatory care that brings providers to people and gives consumers a real voice in decisions of consequence. In individual instances, lessons to avoid as well as to emulate are apparent, but in the final analysis neighborhood health centers have made an important and enduring contribution to health care in the United States.

References

1. Stoeckle, J.D. and Candib, L.M. "The neighborhood health center: reform ideas of yesterday and today," *New England Journal of Medicine* 280:1385-1391, 1969.

2. Schorr, L.B. and English, J.T. "Background, context, and significant issues in neighborhood health center programs," *Milbank Memorial Fund Quarterly* 66 (3, part I):289-296, 1968.

3. Zwick, D.I. "Some accomplishments and findings of neighborhood health centers," *Milbank Memorial Fund Quarterly* 50 (4, part I):387-420, 1972.

4. Hollister, R.M., Kramer, B.M., and Bellin, S.S. "Neighborhood health centers as a social movement." In: Hollister, R.M., Kramer, B.M., and Bellin, S.S. (eds.), *Neighborhood Health Centers.* Lexington Books (D.C. Heath), 1974.

5. Economic Opportunity Act as Amended; 42 USC 2809. The specific authorization for the "Comprehensive Health Services Program" was originally included in 1966 as Section 211-2 and became Section 222(a) (4) through later amendments.

6. Levitan, S.A. "Healing the poor in their back yard." Hollister, R.M., Kramer, B.M., Bellin, S.S. (eds.), *Neighborhood Health Centers.* Lexington, Mass.: Lexington Books, 1974, pp. 51-68.

7. Reynolds, R.A. "Improving access to health care among the poor—the neighborhood health center experience," *Milbank Memorial Fund Quarterly* 54 (1):47-82, 1976.

8. Geiger, H.J. "Community conflict—or community control." Hollister, R.M., Kramer, B.M., and Bellin, S.S. (eds.), *Neighborhood Health Centers.* Lexington, Mass., Lexington Books, pp. 133-142.

9. Caplan, G. *Principles of Preventive Psychiatry.* New York: Basic Books, 1964.

10. Wise, H.B., Torrey, E.F., McDale, A., Perry, G., Bograd, H. "The family health worker," *American Journal of Public Health* 58 (10):1828-1838, 1968.

11. Parker, A.W. The Team Approach to Primary Health Care. Berkeley, California: Neighborhood Health Center Seminar Program, Monograph Series No. 3, January, 1972.

12. Rubin, I.M. and Beckhard, R. "Factors influencing the effectiveness of health teams," *Milbank Memorial Fund Quarterly* 50 (3, part I):317-335, 1972.

13. Bicknell, W.J., Walsh, D.C., and Tanner, M.M. "Substantial or decorative? Physician's assistants and nurse practitioners in the United States," *Lancet* 2:1241-1244, 1974.

14. Olafson, F., Ferguson, A., Jr., and Parker, A.W. Confidentiality: A Guide for Neighborhood Health Centers. Berkeley, California: Neighborhood Health Center Seminar Program, Monograph Series No. 1, 1971.

15. Gordon, J.B. "The politics of community medicine projects: a conflict analysis." In: Hollister, R.M., Kramer, B.M., and Bellin, S.S. (eds.),

Neighborhood Health Centers. Lexington, Mass.: Lexington Books, 1974, pp. 111-122.

16. Macht, L.B. "Neighborhood health centers—perspective on opportunity for comprehensive ambulatory care," *New England Journal of Medicine* 292 (11): 591, 1975.

17. Fein, R. "An economist's view of the neighborhood health center as a new social institution," *Medical Care* 8 (2):104-107, 1970.

18. Bellin, S.S., Geiger, H.J., Gibson, C.D. "Impact of ambulatory health care services on the demand for hospital beds," *New England Journal of Medicine* 280:808-812, 1969.

19. Hillman, B., Charney, E. "A neighborhood health center: what the patients know and think of its operation," *Medical Care* 10 (4):336-344, 1972.

20. Morehead, M.A., Donaldson, R.S., Seravalli, M.R. "Comparisons between OEO neighborhood health centers and other health care providers of ratings of the quality of health care," *American Journal of Public Health* 61:1294-1306, 1971.

21. Ferguson, A.R., The Role of Neighborhood Health Centers in Economic Development. Berkeley, California: Neighborhood Health Center Seminar Program, Monograph Series No. 4, January 1972.

22. Elinson, J. and Herr, C.E.A. "A sociomedical view of neighborhood health centers," *Medical Care* 8 (2):97-103, 1970.

23. Bicknell, W.J. and Walsh, D.C. "Critical experiences in organizing and administering a state certification of need program," *Public Health Reports* 91 (1):29-45, 1976.

24. Home Care Program, East Boston Neighborhood Health Center. Personal communication, Marie Feltin, M.D.

Part II

Neighborhood Psychiatry Program Models

Introduction

This Section includes chapters which describe a number of different program models and experiences of neighborhood practitioners and address specific program and clinical issues in the organization and delivery of neighborhood services. A wide variety of case examples of programs and of client situations are presented to illustrate the conceptual and organizational matters developed in each of the chapters. Throughout, the description reveals a field that is simultaneously spurting in growth and attempting to solve a variety of exceedingly complex dilemmas in service delivery and clinical and community work.

The section begins with a chapter by Reich which serves as a bridge between the last chapter of Part I and what follows in this section. She highlights structural issues in neighborhood health center programs as a context for providing neighborhood mental health services. She further points to problems in service integration within centers and in linkages between neighborhood and backup hospital services as well as with the neighborhood served.

In the chapter by Lowenkopf and Paul, the functions and limitations of a psychiatric consultant in a neighborhood health center are delineated. Problems of access and attempts to integrate the consultant into the center are described. This leads to the subject of the chapter which follows in which a different model of integration of services is developed. Morrill describes this model as the maximum integration of mental health services in a neighborhood health center. He details its evolution and functioning and describes a range of mental health services which are offered, including preventive ones, furthering the discussion of linkages to backup services and to the neighborhood begun by Reich. He also discusses advocacy functions and interstaff relations within a center and focuses on the integration of mental health personnel and services with the center's comprehensive family health care teams. He highlights the advantages of comprehensive services at the neighborhood level and offers the neighborhood health center as ideal provider of mental health services.

Norman follows with a thorough discussion of a program for linking and coordinating neighborhood services—an outreach model penetrating into the grass roots and natural caregiving institutions of the neighborhood. Focusing on how neighborhood services become relevant parts of the neighborhood and its service delivery systems, he describes the potential of neighborhood mental health services for primary prevention and the strengthening of existing neighborhood institutions in their broadest mental health functions. His chapter captures the essences of a major new dimension of neighborhood practice as it evolves beyond the neighborhood health center and into the formal and informal networks of the neighborhood. His discussion of problems of linkage building thus continues those of Reich and Morrill and leads to that offered by Lightfoot, who focuses on linkages to central facilities. Lightfoot raises questions of process, development, and structure in neighborhood services and brings to the fore problems of funding, conflicts, responsibility, and control.

Throughout this section, one sees the emergence (albeit at times problematic) of neighborhood services as primary, first contact, or front-line components of a newly developing mental health delivery system. These services, once viewed as "satellites," emerge as a central element of ambulatory care, with great potential for prevention and for clinical care. Recognition of their twofold need, however, is crucial: to be closely linked to the neighborhood and its formal and informal networks, on the one hand, and to specialized hospital or mental health center based services, on the other. "Neighborhood" and comprehensive neighborhood services thus become a newly evolving arena for mental health practice, building on other work in the field (especially clinical, community, and general hospital liaison psychiatry) but distinctly different in focus, location, content, and conceptualization. We see a beginning reformulation of community mental health practice and the development of a new system of community based service delivery which carries the field beyond the mental health center and more into the community.[a]

---

[a]See also Macht, L.B. "Beyond the Mental Health Center: Planning for a Community of Neighborhoods." *Psychiatric Annals*, 5:7, July, 1975.

6

Conceptual Aspects of Service Integration

Lee Reich

Comprehensive, family-oriented care is usually a goal for those who work in and for a neighborhood health center, but the integration of services required to achieve this challenging goal is not necessarily a solid accomplishment. This chapter makes some observations about the nature of a neighborhood health center as an organization and delineates some of the underlying structural issues which complicate its administrative and clinical functioning. Five years as a clinical psychologist in a health center struggling for internal cohesiveness as well as financial stability convinced this author that some of the difficulties are inherent in the situation of a neighborhood health center, although each event that occurs is experienced by the participants as unique and personal. Examples taken from these experiences at the Neighborhood Family Care Center in Cambridge, Massachusetts serve to illustrate some of the ways in which unresolved structural issues may provide barriers to the integration of services.[a]

Neighborhood health centers of the type organized in the late 1960s under the sponsorship of federal antipoverty programs typically seek to offer coordinated services in neighborhood settings with some degree of consumer input and control. These centers represent an effort to use public funds to give residents of low-income neighborhoods some of the responsibility for services in their communities which are traditionally exercised by lay trustees of large voluntary and public hospitals. In order to accomplish this, representatives of the particular community and of the provider agencies agree on plans for a new organization, involving board, director, and staff, which provide a structure for funding, for administration, and for the professional or clinical direction of a variety of services. Thus, the structure and function of a health center replicates that of a hospital in its essential relationships, yet a neighborhood center faces certain additional challenges because of its special aims. Administrative cooperation between neighborhood residents and professional providers is often complicated by mutual distrust as well as real differences of point of view and of priorities. Clinical coordination of a neighborhood health center usually involves not only a variety of medical services, but

---

[a]Additional perspective was gained through work on the Mental Health Task Force sponsored by the Massachusetts League of Neighborhood Health Centers. This task force assisted in analysing the results of a survey of the mental health programs operating in 19 health centers in the City of Boston in 1973. See also Chapter 11 of this volume.

additional programs such as day care for children, tutoring programs, and other social services. These nonmedical services may be sponsored independently by the health center itself or by other agencies in the community. A neighborhood health center thus involves new and complex collaborations among individuals, groups, and agencies, many of whom have never been part of the same institution.

Issues of Organizational Coordination and Linkages

Despite the bewildering variety, which at first makes every center seem unique, certain underlying organizational problems must be approached and solved simultaneously if a center is to fulfill its purpose. Thus, the key relationships are between the health center and the community, between the health center and its backup institutions and, within the health center, among the various services. The administrative and clinical coordination of services obviously depends upon both the fiscal and administrative provisions linking the health center to the local community and the working relationships with backup institutions. In order to understand the organizational stresses which may create barriers to the integration of services, each of these relationships is considered in more detail.

Consumer input is usually exercised through a policy or advisory board in conjunction with an administrator responsible to that board. Centers vary greatly in their sources of funding and in the amount of control the neighborhood board and nonmedical administrator have over medical services. However, all administrative matters, such as hiring of personnel, program priorities, purchasing, the allocation of space, and so forth, have profound clinical implications, and the functioning of the center director and the board of directors has direct impact on the operation of the center. This impact sometimes involves tension and strife, yet it is an essential part of the mechanism through which a center is responsive to the community it serves.

Because of the need for medical and mental health backup, the "outpost" health center is inextricably a part of the existing delivery system at the same time that it represents an effort to change that system and to add other elements to it. The medical service units within a health center usually duplicate the departmental structure of a hospital, and the neighborhood center is structurally linked to a backup institution through staff appointments which provide a chain of clinical responsibility and through a system for referrals and consultation. Thus, the clinical services offered by a health center are organized on the basis of the traditional medical specialities—pediatrics, adult medicine, psychiatry or mental health, and so forth. Social service may or may not be a separate unit, and centers also vary in how they provide obstetrical care and gynecological services. Unless the hospital departments are themselves coordinated through programs in community medicine or primary care, the coordination and cooperation necessary for family-oriented or "whole-person" care must come primarily from relationships and arrangements within the health center.

A significant modification of traditional patterns of health care has occurred through the development of new kinds of caregivers. The use of nurse practitioners and the development of career ladders for paraprofessionals in the fields of health, mental health, and social service has been a rewarding and successful part of many health centers. However, such delegation of medical and other kinds of professional responsibility adds to the complexity of the clinical authority structure within a health center as a part of a larger health system.

Clinical and administrative coordination are likely to be further complicated by the fact that a variety of services in additon to medical care may be sponsored by the center. Backup and professional supervision may be provided separately for the several component units of a neighborhood center. For this reason the relationship of mental health services to other components may be very complex. The comprehensive mental health center which provides backup and validation for mental health services at the outpost center is basically a separate institution from the medical backup system, although a hospital department of psychiatry may be part of both systems. This separation of mental health from the medical system creates an inside-outside problem for mental health staff, regardless of whether their primary allegiance is to the health center or to the backup mental health facility. Mental health staff are either consultants to the health center or they belong to the health center staff and are not an integral part of the larger mental health center. Basic questions to be asked are: Where do mental health staff really identify? What agency commands their primary loyalty? To whose clinical and administrative authority are they subject and under what circumstances? Programs sponsored directly by the health center or those relating to other agencies, such as the Visiting Nurse Association, may face similar issues in relation to medical services or to the administrative structure of a health center.

Within any particular center the integration of services takes place in both formal and informal ways. A neighborhood health center usually fosters close, personal interaction among staff members of various units, but centers, like hospitals, vary greatly in the degree of structural integration of various kinds of service. Some have a medical director who is responsible to some but not necessarily all service units, as well as to both the backup medical facility and the administrative structure of the neighborhood center. In other centers the head of each service unit works with the center administrator and the backup facility. In understanding the structure of any given center, the crucial questions are how medical responsibility, program coordination, and service leadership are exercised and how clinical authority relates to administrative authority and to the backup institutions. In answering such questions, one must look at the lines of communication and chains of authority and responsibility for any given employee and determine who can hire and who can fire employees and how they are paid.

Interaction Among Organizations, Systems, and Components

Having reviewed the components of a typical health center, the organizational nature of a neighborhood health center can be described more accurately. It may be seen as being, of necessity, an incomplete merger of several systems. In one sense, the initial structure of a health center is a kind of contract between various interested parties who agree to work together. Some working rules and operating agreements are made at the time the neighborhood health center is created, and these are embodied in the initial administrative powers given to the center director by its various components. All functions and powers, however, are not merged, and an important element in any center is the agreement to collaborate on an ongoing basis. A single decision-making process or clear-cut hierarchical authority structure does not, therefore, exist. Rather, negotiation and consensus building become an important part of the administration, and problems and misunderstandings are unavoidable.

The nature of the initial working agreement—the structural arrangements among the various components—is likely to be an important factor in determining the course of subsequent development. Relationships among the components of a health center as established in its initial organization may be vague or to some extent in conflict. Centers vary enormously in the degree of centralization of administrative powers and in the complexity of the lines of clinical responsibility within the center and in linking the center to its backup facilities. In addition, participants in a health center may have different views of the original agreement, and as individuals come and go, perceptions and patterns of interaction also change. Thus, many problems must be faced in daily operations and development continues as the center functions, but the process may be slow and difficult.

The complex collaboration typical of a health center, where many diverging needs and perceptions must be dealt with, places a great burden on the individuals involved. Conflicts between one kind of service and another, or tensions among representatives of the community, or between the center and the backup institutions are often viewed as personality clashes when, in part, they represent unresolved structural issues. The various power structures involved seem destined to clash, and the resulting confusion and tension are disturbing to all participants. Nevertheless, these confrontations offer an opportunity to encompass new points of view and to learn to function in different ways.

Case Illustration

The Neighborhood Family Care Center in Cambridge, Massachusetts, is an instance of a health center in which the initial working agreement between representatives of the community and the participating professional agencies was relatively vague and limited, and much was left to be negotiated as the center grew. Conflict involving board, administrator, staff, and participating agencies and institutions resulted, as well as a high staff turnover as changes and reorganization occurred. As a place to work and grow professionally and personally, it was tumultuous, but deeply rewarding. The story of this health center cannot accurately be told from any one point of view, but some aspects of its initial structure and its history may be singled out in order to illustrate the influence of structural arrangements upon efforts to provide coordinated services.

The Neighborhood Family Care Center began in 1968 as the Experimental Service Delivery System with the following aims: (1) to coordinate the delivery to a specified neighborhood of health and social services; (2) to provide health care in a neighborhood setting; and (3) to deliver health care in a manner that was accountable to the community. Community representatives participated in the planning from the outset in cooperation with representatives of four Cambridge agencies: the Cambridge Department of Health and Hospitals, Cambridge Family Counseling Service, the Cambridge Mental Health Association, and the Alliance of Cambridge Settlement Houses. Health care and social services were to be provided "under one roof" in a building obtained through the cooperation of the Massachusetts Institute of Technology. Community "control" was to be exercised through a Joint Policy Board on which the majority of seats were to be held by residents of the area served, but the cooperating agencies were represented by one member each. The administrator of the center was to be hired directly by the Board, but staff worked under a variety of arrangements. Medical services, initially pediatrics but later including adult medicine, obstetrics, and gynecology, were provided on an in-kind basis by The Cambridge Hospital. Clinics were staffed primarily by nurse practitioners who were hired through the hospital and were medically responsible to their respective medical departments and the hospital and health department nursing services. Social workers, and later a group worker and a psychologist, were hired on a contract basis from the cooperating agencies using federal and privately granted funds. For administrative matters, social service and mental health staff were responsible to the Director and ultimately to the Board of the Center, but responsibility for professional supervision rested not in the Center but with the respective outside agencies. Eventually paraprofessional workers were hired for drug programs and other activities, and these workers were responsible only to the Center Director.

The organizational structure of the Neighborhood Family Care Center as initially established consisted of small service units, each with separate arrangements for clinical backup and with decision-making authority, in some instances clearly resting in the backup hospital rather than with Center staff. At no time was there a medical director—that is, a physician with jurisdiction across service units—whether paid by the health center or by the backup hospital. The absence of a medical director reflected not only the fragmentation of professional services but also the widely held conception among the neighborhood residents that they "controlled" the Center on the basis of administrative powers alone. Unfortunately, despite sincere efforts by all concerned, conflicts continued and the various participants in the Center came to have increasingly divergent views as to the proper powers and functions of the Board and the director.

A limited step toward functional coordination of services occurred when a psychiatrist, long dedicated to neighborhood-based services, was appointed as Director of Clinical Services. Although he had direct medical responsibility only for the mental health staff (psychiatric residents and the clinical psychologist), he was nevertheless known and respected by the chiefs of the hospital's departments of pediatrics and adult medicine and by the neighborhood board, and he was empowered to act as a consultant to all staff and to the directors of the Center, serving as a negotiator to some extent when crises arose.

A few concrete examples point out the impact of the fragmented clinical structure which characterized the Neighborhood Family Care Center. A variety of efforts were made by Center administrators and staff to provide for program coordination and integration of services to clients. Time was set aside for a staff meeting; and under the leadership of the Director of Clinical Services, the staff was organized at one time into two interdisciplinary teams which met on a weekly basis. These meetings were in essence social service or mental health conferences. Schedulaing difficulties consistently presented a major obstacle to interdisciplinary meetings. Fixed clinic times and other staff commitments made it very difficult to find times for case conferences or team meetings, and neither the administrator nor the Director of Clinical Services had authority to rearrange clinics or to adjust priorities for the medical staff.

Eventually, a variety of problems combined to undercut the usefulness of interdisciplinary teams; and no further steps were taken at an organizational level to provide for the integration of services. The basic separateness of the adult and the pediatric clinics is reflected in the fact that following the demise of teams, the mental health/social service staff came to meet with the pediatric nurse practitioners in their office for one lunch meeting and with the nurses for the adult clinics on another day in their clinic office. However, personal relationships among staff of all kinds remained warm and cooperative and individuals continued to collaborate around the needs of particular families through all the vicissitudes of the health care center itself.

Thus, the initial working agreement creating the health center which came to be called the Neighborhood Family Care Center was incomplete. A variety of services were housed "under one roof." Some provision was made for administrative coordination, but there was no structural provision in the initial working agreement for real clinical coordination and planning. This situation never changed, and the lack of a clinical director empowered by all participants to function within the center placed a great burden on the administrator on the one hand and on the staff on the other. While other factors, such as persistent and serious funding problems, undoubtedly influenced the functioning of this center, unresolved structural conflicts were central in a process which eventually resulted in the gradual suspension of the clinical programs of the Center.

Conclusions

The coordination of health care and other kinds of services within a neighborhood center depends heavily on the administrative structure of the center itself and also on the effectiveness of the organization of each service unit. The number of complex relationships and new patterns of interaction which must be handled by the board, administration, and staff of a health center foster conflict and frustration as symptoms of the stress of these new patterns. But stress is inevitable when growth and change are taking place, and such conflicts and frustrations can serve as catalysts for constructive developments, if the existing structure can respond adequately. Interdisciplinary cooperation does not happen automatically and must overcome many obstacles. Services of all kinds, however, may be enriched by the opportunity to work together and to learn from the members of the community which is served.

7

The Role of the Psychiatric Consultant in a Neighborhood Health Center

Eugene L. Lowenkopf and
Diana Paul

This chapter reports the experience of a group of psychiatric consultants working in a variety of roles over a five-and-a-half-year period at a neighborhood health center. It describes the development of a division of mental health at the center, and follows its history and evolution with some consideration given to the problems that have arisen.

Background: Initial Organization and Personnel

In July, 1966, Montefiore Hospital in the Bronx, New York City, received funding from the Office of Economic Opportunity to establish a neighborhood health center which was mandated to provide high-quality ambulatory health care to the residents of its catchment area. At that time, the area contained 8,000 residents, mostly of Puerto Rican origin, with some blacks and some elderly whites. All statistics for the area indicated that, from a health viewpoint, it was one of the poorest and most disadvantaged in the city. The catchment area has subsequently been greatly expanded to include about 45,000 residents, and the percentage of blacks has increased markedly, but the same social and health indices pertain. At the time of its founding, the center, as a pilot program, was called the Neighborhood Medical Care Demonstration, but it is now the Dr. Martin Luther King, Jr., Health Center.

To fulfill its mandate in an area with virtually no health resources conveniently available to its population, the immediate problems were to establish a physical location for health services and to develop a group of people who could provide such services. A location was found quickly enough and a storefront health center was opened. A core staff of committed and dedicated professionals was available at Montefiore Hospital, but it was clear that they could not provide the wide variety of social and legal as well as medical services that was required. Because neighborhood residents could fulfill certain functions, a training program of some size was developed which provided for an analysis of the functions performed by health professionals and a restructuring of responsibility leading to a team approach to delivery of health care.

The health team at King is the basic unit for providing services, each team being assigned the care of all people living in a designated number of blocks. "Care" refers to direct medical services as well as to other forms of assistance that lead to improved health, such as obtaining sufficient heat in winter and adequate welfare

payments. The team consists of a public health nurse, several family health workers, an internist, a pediatrician, and a lawyer. In addition to their specific professional training, the nurse, physicians, and lawyer have had courses orienting
them to the community and to social medicine before they begin work at the
center; they reside, for the most part, outside of the area.

The family health workers, who reside in the community and are "nonprofessionals," are usually women, some of whom have not graduated from high
school. They have trained for twenty-four weeks in home nursing skills, welfare
law, health education, and social advocacy. They are frequent visitors to the
homes of their patients where they perform nursing functions, such as taking
blood pressures and pulse rates, checking the urine of diabetics, giving enemas,
and instructing the families in health matters. Each reports daily to her supervising nurse who directs what she does and occasionally visits the patients herself. The nurse is also responsible for seeing that the patients visit their physicians during clinic hours at the center. Doctors work primarily at the Center
and in affiliated hospitals.

The team obviously relies on its nonprofessionals to assist a limited number
of professionals in providing broader health care services. Once weekly, it meets
to discuss problem families or households. At these sessions, which the nurse
leads, the family health worker presents the case and the problems, and the
nurse uses all the available expertise to determine how to help the family. These
team conferences serve not only as problem-solving sessions but also as training
grounds for the staff.

This somewhat simplified description of who does what and how the team
operates evolved over the first two years of the Center's functioning, and has
remained essentially the same in spite of a variety of organizational and administrative changes.

Development of Mental Health Services: The Team and
the Psychiatrist

In the original planning of the center, no provision was made for psychiatric
staffing or services, despite the center's objective of providing family-oriented
health care with concern for the psychological well being of the patient. And
despite the enthusiasm and dedication of the original staff working out of the
storefront, considerable difficulties arose in just this area. More often than not,
the patient or family presented in team conference proved to have serious
psychological problems which could not be helped by anyone at the meeting.
A strong need was felt by all the staff for additional psychiatric information
and recommendations.

At just about this time, in January 1968, the King Center catchment area
was made part of the catchment area of Bronx State Hospital. This provided

many advantages to the Center; whereas formerly patients from the area who required psychiatric hospitalization were taken to a city hospital ten miles away and then to a state hospital thirty miles away, such patients could now be hospitalized five miles from their homes and could begin definitive treatment sooner rather than later. Liaison arrangements for aftercare could also be made more efficiently, and a psychiatric staff from the hospital was available to consult on patients.

Initially, patients were brought from the Center to the hospital to be interviewed by a psychiatrist or a psychologist on the hospital geographic unit serving the King area. Following this interview, recommendations for treatment and follow up were made to the team. Information flow in both directions was communicated through the Center's liaison worker, a nonprofessional. Although this program was satisfactory from the point of view of taking care of problem patients, it only provided a limited amount of instruction to the team. It also did not expose the hospital staff to the community and milieu in which the patient lived, nor to the people who were to carry out its recommendations.

One other circumstance led to a change in the locus of consultations: the obvious tension had developed in some teams among the various professionals and nonprofessionals. Problems concerning role definition, areas of responsibility and authority, racism, and disagreements concerning medical ethics, were becoming apparent in the team and often found their expression in the soft area of psychiatric management rather than in the more clear-cut areas of medicine and pediatrics. Because of this tension it was felt that psychiatric consultation should occur in a team conference setting where the consultant could perform a group process function, in addition to providing patient information.

Consequently, in the summer of 1968, when the catchment population expanded from 8,000 to 45,000, and the center moved from the storefront to a large, well-equipped remodeled warehouse, the nature of the psychiatric consultation changed. Each of several consultants from the state hospital was assigned to work with a team for a half day a week; part of this time was spent at the team meeting and the remainder was spent interviewing patients directly in the presence of the referring team member. The functions of the mental health professional were primarily team teaching and consultation, supervising the staff on their long-term efforts with patients rather than attempting any direct long-term treatment, although in addition to their responsibilities to the team, some of the consultants were involved in other teaching, research, supervisory and planning capacities.

Of all the team members, the family health worker enters the home most frequently and is most quickly drawn into the dynamics of the family; her work suffers most if she does not appreciate the psychological role thrust upon her. On the other hand, as the worker closest to the family and usually of the same ethnic group, she has probably the greatest potential for effective communication. In the original planning, extensive use of this group of workers was envisioned for carrying out a considerable amount of the mental health work at the Center. Consequently, a training program for them was begun; it consisted of twelve weekly one-and-one-half hour seminars and concentrated on the recognition, understanding, and handling of psychiatric problems, on personality development, and on treatment modalities. Little emphasis was placed on formal diagnosis or inpatient treatment, but there was emphasis on the situations that precipitate decompensation, the factors that influence recovery, and the problems in living that the psychiatric patient faces. These seminars were intended to complement and place in an organized framework the clinical material to which the worker was exposed daily. However, despite original hopes, the family health workers were not, as a group, interested in general principles or theory and most were only interested in the very specific and immediate problems that their patients presented.

At a later time, a great deal of interest was expressed by the supervising nursing staff in having some formal training in psychiatry, particularly as related to the complex of social, economic, and psychological problems seen in patients in this community. When this request was met and case material was discussed, only the nurse who presented was interested; when more general theory was discussed, the attendance dropped. Then a very specific request arose for training in psychopharmacology; when this was complied with, attendance dropped further. Discussion with a number of nurses, as well as the nursing director, suggested that nurses primarily wanted help with problem-solving and reassurance, and that these were best rendered on an individual basis, not in a group forum. A course in psychopharmacology for the physicians at the Center met with little more success, although individual physicians, over a period of years, have requested supervision with their difficult patients.

These negative experiences with formal training programs, at the hands of several teachers with different viewpoints and different techniques, led us to conclude that teaching efforts should be exclusively through team conferences and patient practice.

In formulating the role of a psychiatric consultant in a team, a model team had been postualted. In this team, each individual would function with a clear picture of his own role and how he related to each other team member and to patients. Leadership would be in the hands of the nurse, and problems presented to the consultant would be clearly phrased and in the consultant's own sphere of knowledge. His opinion would be eagerly sought and his advice immediately acted upon. It was anticipated that some problems would arise between individual members of the team and, in these cases, the psychiatrist would promote greater effectiveness by helping the individuals concerned to understand each other better. It quickly became apparent that this prediction was unduly optimistic and problems arose in many areas. These included team organization, personal difficulties of the individual members of the medical team, community attitudes toward psychiatry, difficulties separating psychiatric problems from the social and economic problems with which they are often associated, and inadequate preparation of the consultants for team and community work.

The most serious problems in team organization concerned the question of leadership, the role alteration of the various team members, and the ambiguous position of the consultants. Although frequent statements were made that the public health nurse was the coordinator of the team functioning, she constantly deferred to medical opinions, even in legal or social matters. Nurses were also unsure whether their supervision of the family health workers should consist of directing them or advising them. Family health workers, for their part, were anxious in their new professional roles and alternated between seeing themselves as spokesmen for the community and its goals, and identifying with the professional staff and its goals; the two were not always the same. They often doubted if they had anything special to offer, and needed clear statements of what contributions they made toward accomplishing the objectives of the center. Physicians tended to assume leadership in all areas and to minimize the importance of social and cultural factors.

When the psychiatric consultant appeared at the conference of a team struggling with problems of direction and leadership, he was often received with confusion and his role was unclear. He was frequently seen as the agent of the center's administration and, therefore, either a potential leader or an interloper who would report back the weaknesses of the team. Some of these problems were resolved with the passage of time while others, despite much effort, continued to plague consultants and teams.

Case Illustrations

Several examples of cases presented at conferences follow which illustrate how the team functioned, how the psychiatrist was utilized, what kinds of problems in consultation arose, and what sorts of treatment recommendations were made.

Case I

A family was presented in which the mother, a 29-year-old woman, had on a number of occasions been hospitalized in state institutions with a diagnosis of chronic schizophrenia. She was not living with her four children and her invalid mother and often disappeared overnight. Arrangements had already been made for welfare assistance and a part-time homemaker, but the children were presenting problems in school and the grandmother felt she could no longer cope with them.

The team was perplexed concerning what steps to take, and the psychiatrist suggested that the role of the grandmother be strengthened by the family health worker. No one on the team responded to the suggestion during the conference and one of the family health workers condemned the mother for exploiting welfare. The nurse agreed and suggested that welfare be stopped so that the mother would be forced either to go to work or starve. The internist suggested that the children's problem would be solved if they were placed in an institution and the family broken up. Further discussion was dropped at this point but some weeks later the family health worker reported to the psychiatrist that she had been advising the grandmother to set limits and to make the children participate in the housework; they had begun to settle down in school, and the family situation was quieter.

Case II

In another team, a family health worker presented a family who was taking care of an elderly aunt while her son was in prison. The old woman was confused and incontinent, but the family wanted to keep its promise to her son to care for and not hospitalize her. When the psychiatrist reviewed the alternatives and underlined the poor prognosis, the family health worker burst into tears. She said that she could not return to the family with such a bad report and would rather quit; she then questioned the competence of the psychiatrist. The other family health workers were also dismayed at the psychiatrist's inability to do anything, but then began to tell the presenting worker that she just couldn't face the fact that nothing could be done to improve the patient's psychiatric state. The family health worker realized her involvement and was able to help the family plan more realistically for the patient.

Case III

In a third example, a sensitive young family health worker presented the case of a young mother who was dying of cancer of the cervix. The patient had several children who were currently being looked after by her mother. The family health worker blamed the imminent death on sloppy diagnosis and poor treatment at the local city hospital. She did not know what to do concerning the dying patient and did not know how to talk to the patient's mother or to the children. Here the consultant discussed with the team their feelings about death, following which the internist talked about the natural history of cancer of the cervix. The team then formulated recommendations which the family health worker could carry out.

Discussion: Accomplishments and Problems

These cases give some idea of the problems that arose in the team and how the psychiatric consultants handled them. In each of these cases some constructive suggestions were made which would, with the help of an informed team, be carried out to a greater or lesser extent. Much, however, could not be changed readily, such as judgmental attitudes toward patients, denial of mental illness, readiness to abandon problem patients, reluctance to accept realistic limitations, hostility to psychiatry, and difficulty being objective toward patients.

The major thrust of the consultants' efforts has been in working with teams handling problem households; originally no provision had been made for treatment of special groups of patients such as alcoholics and addicts, and children and adolescents. In each of the two areas of substance abuse, a nonprofessional specialist was appointed to coordinate case finding, referral to other agencies, and long-term follow-up; although a psychiatrist was available to the coordinator as a consultant, the coordinator functioned essentially on his own. Both the alcohol and the narcotics coordinators were former drug abusers, and were well acquainted with available community resources and methods of treatment.

Just as a consultant relationship had been worked out with Bronx State Hospital for help to the adult patients, a similar arrangement was developed with the Bronx Children's Hospital to provide for evaluations and treatment recommendations for disturbed youngsters. In view of the limited number of available child psychiatrists, they were not assigned to teams but saw patients only in the presence of team members. Their consultations served not only as a direct patient service, but as staff education as well.

During the first two years of its history, the team consultation program seemed to work well; many patients were seen and many treatment recommendations carried out. The teams seemed to be learning from the consultants, and the nature of the requests for assistance were becoming more sophisticated. There was a general feeling of satisfaction on the part of both the center and consultant staffs, although in some teams certain seemingly insoluble problems arose. In one team, for example, a conflict arose for the consultant between his wish to do what he felt was right for the patient and his satisfying the team's wishes. In this case, he refused to sign papers requesting that a child be taken from his home and placed in foster care. The consultant explained his reasoning to the team, which had already taken steps to arrange the placement. A nurse who was, on this occasion, the team's spokesman, disagreed strongly, criticized the consultant's competence, and stopped referring patients to him, while further attempting to have the child placed away from home. The consultant appealed to his superiors and to administration for assistance, but unfortunately this did not lead to a reexamination of roles and pruposes.

In another team, a power struggle developed between the consultant and the team concerning the presence of a visiting medical student at the team conference. The psychiatrist felt that the team conference served a useful teaching purpose and should be open to selected visitors; this was indeed a policy of the center which functioned as a demonstration program. The team stated that only visitors who had something special to contribute should be permitted to attend conferences; team members also questioned whether the students would maintain confidentiality. This episode occurred at a time when the team was undergoing a period of self-criticism and doubt, and it is quite possible that visitors would have been better tolerated at other times. As a result of this conflict, the psychiatrist left the team. Again, superiors and administration did not attempt a reconciliation.

These conflicts which were not resolved except by the psychiatrist's departure from the teams created a feeling of impotence on the part of other consultants as well. All consultants felt that without a full-time chief of their own at the center they lacked a voice in determination of policy, and could not affect the ways in which their services could be utilized. The Center administration, on the other hand, felt that consultants did not sense the problems of the groups they were meant to assist, and lacked skill in carrying out their mission.

Although it is difficult even now to determine the exact causes of the conflicts, it does seem that one major problem was the assumption of the role of ombudsman by the consultants. Many team members resented the consultant's involvement in their interpersonal problems and felt he was overstepping his bounds, even when they respected his ability with patients. The team, as has already been pointed out, had many difficult issues to work out from the time of its inception, and just as these prblems had previously expressed themselves in the area of mental health, they continued to do so. The consultant had limited power to effect change and, by becoming involved in interpersonal rather than clinical issues, tended to weaken his role as teacher.

With a somewhat reduced number of consultants, the luxury of having one consultant to each team was no longer possible. The administration requested that consultants take referrals in rotation and discontinue entirely their role as team consultants. The psychiatric staff felt that not being related to a single team would seriously compromise its teaching role by preventing continuity of contact and presented some alternative plans. These were overruled by the administration, further convincing the psychiatric staff of its impotence, and more defections occurred.

Fortunately for the Center, other potential sources of consultants existed in the various programs of the Albert Einstein College of Medicine Department of Psychiatry. Each of these programs had its own agenda, such as the training of medical students or of fellows, and the Center had to work out arrangements whereby these borrowed staffs could fulfill their academic responsibilities as well as see patients. Conflicts that resulted have posed problems, and some of these programs have discontinued their contacts with the Center.

Some of the resulting slack in terms of patient care has been taken up by the hiring of a part-time psychiatrist who works for the center. At present he provides the bulk of direct patient consultation, although some patients are seen by other consultants who have remained. Child and adolescent consultation programs continue with staff from the Bronx Children's Hospital. The narcotics and alcohol programs also continue, but without psychiatric supervision. A training program for family health workers also exists in which they can participate with medical students in the intensive work-up of selected cases; because not all workers are interested, only a limited number are invited to join.

Conclusions

Retrospectively, this experience reveals that much has been accomplished despite some major difficulties. Original doubts as to whether mental health services could be delivered in a neighborhood health center rather than in a purely psychiatric community mental health center and whether it was a good idea to do so have been dispelled. The examples given, as well as innumerable similar ones, demonstrate that people can be reached and meaningful services can be delivered at such an agency. It is important to bear in mind, though, that mental health is not the primary reason for the existence of the neighborhood health center and mental health services must compete with other more tangible services for the interest and time of the staff. The unpalatable truths that our needs and programs will often take second or third order priority and that we will not always have an active voice in policy determination must also be recognized. In addition, work in this area will often take place with people who are antagonistic to and frightened by psychiatry, and our work will not always be respected or appreciated.

Recognizing these givens, we should devote ourselves to direct patient care and to case-related supervision of interested staff, and should avoid a nonspecific role, such as general troubleshooter. We should also insist upon representation in the policy-making councils of the organization, at least to the extent that we help to determine how best to deliver our services. Failure to do so can only lead to time-consuming, nonproductive conflict and demoralization.

8

Integration of Mental Health and Comprehensive Health Services in a Neighborhood Health Center

Richard G. Morrill

This chapter presents the experience of a mental health program's first six years in a comprehensive neighborhood health center. The current revolution in decentralized primary health care delivery in the neighborhood has been largely ignored by mental health practitioners who often seem secure in their separate community mental health center, relying too heavily on medical school stereotypes to relate to the rest of the health care professions. Neighborhood programs and health centers have had very low priority in their thinking. Conceptually, they have not yet become a possibility for many of our program planners.

The intent of this chapter is to present both the advantages for mental health delivery in working through a neighborhood primary health care system and a frank appraisal of one attempt to adapt to the unique opportunities of such a system. The major focus here will not be on program facets we are proud of, such as our community board, our paraprofessionals from the community, our specific therapeutic approaches; these are also found in other programs. Instead, the focus will be on phenomena which usually represent "the forest which can't be seen for the trees", that is, the comprehensive neighborhood health center system we work through and our attempts to get "inside" it to improve the effectiveness of our mental health services.

Background

A large variety of programs and funding sources are subsumed under the term "neighborhood health center". These have included health centers with various degrees of comprehensiveness funded by such sources as OEO and Model Cities (before 1974), municipal governments, Maternal and Infant Care funding, private hospitals, HEW, third-party payments (Medicaid, Medicare, Blue Cross-Blue Shield, and private health insurance), and prepaid health maintenance organizations. Despite the diversity of sources, they often share elements common to comprehensive services delivered through group settings in decentralized sites with some degree of consumer control. The inclusion of mental health services in these has been advocated by Goldensohn [1,2] on the basis of his experience with the Health Insurance Plan of New York and Gibson [3] on a theoretical basis. After sharing our experiences on mental health delivery with a number of these programs informally, we feel that the findings in this chapter

can have value for general applicability, with modifications for the setting and
its constraints.

The Setting

Roxbury Comprehensive Community Health Center (RCCHC) is an HEW 314e-
funded neighborhood health center serving 42,000 people in Boston's black and
Puerto Rican community. It is operated by a community board elected in an
open election in Roxbury's stores and churches. The health center has separated
from its parent Boston University Medical Center (peacefully), is incorporated,
and receives its grant directly from HEW, while maintaining an affiliation with
Boston University Medical Center as its backup. Current services at the health
center include: internal medicine, pediatrics, mental health, gynecology, social
services, nursing, community health workers, dentistry, dietetics, and laboratory; it also contains a full X-ray unit and pharmacy. Staff members work as
two health care teams, each of which meets weekly to discuss families and
patient care issues, and each of the clinical disciplines represented is active on
each team. Internists, pediatricians, and nurse practitioners serve as primary
care staff. Unregistered walk-in patients are seen in a special triage clinic and
then followed up by one of the health care teams for ongoing care.
       The mental health program described in this chapter has been designed for
maximum integration into the health center, rather than as a special clinic
within the program. A full-time senior mental health staff member functions as
the mental health supervisor on each of the health care teams with two mental
health staff members. The disciplines include psychiatry, psychology, psychiatric social work, psychiatric nursing, and paraprofessionals from the community
health worker department. These staff members offer a full range of mental
health consultation, education, evaluation, and therapies, with referral mainly
from the health care team but also by direct request from patients. Second
priority is given to referrals from outside agencies.
       Both adults and children are seen and all the services are family oriented.
Children needing specialized assessments or extended therapy are referred to
the backup Solomon C. Fuller Community Mental Health and Retardation
Center. The Fuller CMHC also provides a consultant for a special child diagnostic conference each week and provides links for day hospital, inpatient, and
drug and alcohol programs.
       Patient referrals are seen by mental health staff within a few days — often
on the same day if the patient is at the health center. Both the mental health
and social service departments present all evaluations in a joint intake conference which formulates a plan and sets a follow-up date. Many of the
families are also discussed with other health care providers informally and in the
health care team meeting.

Special projects include an activities group for aftercare patients from the state mental hospital, an aftercare seminar to help other health care staff follow these patients, a project to evaluate and treat stress in hypertensive patients, several groups, and an interdisciplinary child advocacy team which attempts to provide early evaluation and alternatives to separation for potential child neglect and abuse cases.

If the comprehensive neighborhood health center offers unique advantages for mental health programs, how can these programs be introduced into a health center to maximize its potential? The mental health program which began at RCCHC six years ago attempted to apply certain principles derived from experience in other health centers and community settings to make its service more appropriate and effective in this type of subsystem [4,5,6,7]. This chapter will review those principles and compare their intention with what was observed over the past six years in the areas of patient accessibility, range of mental health services, interstaff relationships, family health care teams, relationship to the neighborhood health center as a system of health care, and relationship to the backup community mental health center.

Patient Accessibility

In 1970 it was felt that what mental health had to offer was usually inaccessible, not only because of physical distance (from institutions) but also of psychological distance (the stigma of "crazy houses" and "psycho clinics"), and that location in a neighborhood health center would improve this situation.

In 1976 the general consensus among staff and patients who have had contact with different mental health settings is that the services at RCCHC are much more accessible and acceptable. For example, the natural family atmosphere that pervades the waiting room where adults and children come for a variety of services decreases the strangeness and awkwardness felt by people who have not been socialized into psychiatric patienthood. Housing the mental health staff in the same area as the general health care staff has also been very important; they are thus seen as an integral part of the health center. Further, the setting in a local neighborhood allows staff to relate to neighborhood life — helping block clubs, being a part of the community grapevine, and hearing much sooner about consumer likes and dislikes regarding services and personnel. One indication of this has been an increasing number of mental health referrals by friends or family. Because the mental health staff do not rotate, the opportunity exists to know patients and families over a period of time, giving staff a longitudinal view of mental illness. Opportunity exists for continuing intervention, if needed in crisis situations, because a trusting relationship has been built, not too dissimilar from that of the old-time general practitioner who became a friend of the family and through his closer relationship became much more effective in the areas of primary and secondary prevention.

An example illustrates how the neighborhood health center setting can facilitate treatment.

A 47-year-old divorced mother of five who was isolated, extremely sensitive to rejection from others, and subject to recurrent severe depression, dropped out of group treatment at the health center after she had become very angry at the therapist who, she felt, had demeaned her. She subsequently failed to respond to letters or calls offering her a chance to return and discuss it. One year later, while sitting in the waiting room for an appointment with another doctor, her former therapist walked by and waved warmly. She called the next week and asked for an appointment, stating that she had been on the verge of suicide and needed help. Later she explained that her pride could not let her return for help, but the friendly attitude of the therapist, who she had seen quite by accident in the waiting room, caused her to doubt her original perception that he was angry at her and made it possible for her to call again.

This illustrates one benefit of practicing in a physical setting that draws a wide range of people with different needs.

Some indication of patient attitudes toward obtaining mental health services at the center was shown by an informal survey of patients in the waiting room selected at random. Most of those approached did not know that mental health services were a part of the program. (This is not surprising since there had been no special effort made to publicize these services at the center.) However, when the patients were asked where they would first turn if mental illness occurred in their family, they nearly unanimously replied, "the RCCHC," because they could trust them to find a good psychiatrist. This underscores the importance of delivering mental health services through an organization which can establish basic trust with the consumer. Simply to have mental health staff present in such a health center, however, is not enough. Equally important is the way they function with the health center's staff.

Range of Mental Health Services

In 1970, at the outset of the program, it was felt that RCCHC should offer the complete range of ambulatory mental health services — consultation, treatment, and mental health education in a neighborhood setting by a staff of professionals and paraprofessionals. This attempt was guided by the belief that these services would be more effective in a neighborhood health program and that the poor had long been deprived of them — psychiatric *treatment* being provided for suburbs, psychiatric *consultation* for the "inner city."

By 1976, the full range of mental health consultation, education, and ambulatory treatment services had been provided, including diagnostic evaluation;

a variety of therapies, including crisis, short-term, long-term insight (limited), group, family, and drug; supportive aftercare; and certain child psychiatric services. Staff had devoted approximately 70 percent of their clinical time to direct services and 30 percent to indirect consultation with other staff. Program consultation with other agencies in the community was largely carried out by the local community mental health center consultation and education team.

In contrast to the expectations of many psychiatrists, experience has provided evidence that the poor and minorities *can* make good use of insight psychotherapy, depending, as in all groups, on the individual; the meaning and impact of self-discovery about one's interpersonal functioning is not limited to class or race. The fact that the mental health staff are full time and continuous at the Neighborhood Health Center has allowed them to tailor insight psychotherapy to the individual, sometimes proceeding on a nontraditional basis. For example, instead of therapy simply ending if the patient drops out after a particular crisis has subsided, he may be encouraged to return during subsequent difficulties. A continuous thread of insight is maintained between the mental health staff member and the patient so that he or she can resume treatment even after a time lapse of some months.

In RCCHC and other neighborhood health centers, experience demonstrates that both staff consultation and direct patient services must be included for effective mental health staff functioning. Mental health staff lose credibility with other staff when they only *talk* about patients and do not *see* them directly. Direct services are the "stock in trade" of the NHC, and the staff can not ignore this if they are to be relevant. On the other hand, mental health staff who do not offer consultation to other staff on the emotional aspects of their patients or coordinate their care for a family are not utilizing the center setting for maximum benefit as a mental health tool and could just as well be practicing elsewhere. The necessary balance between the direct and indirect work in a health center is made difficult by several factors: increasing reliance on third-party payments which support direct patient care only; health directors or administrators who cannot "see" the less visible results of helping a patient *through* another staff member when clinically indicated; other disciplines which carry on ongoing, unrecognized mental health roles with their patients but find it difficult to ask for mental health consultation to improve their skills; and some health planners who feel that quality mental health services can only be provided by psychiatrists.

Mental health treatment and preventive approaches which have worked especially well in the program at the RCCHC have included:

Family Therapy. This has been a "natural" for the program because families are already involved in the health center through their use of the comprehensive services and do not have to be pulled into a setting with which they are unfamiliar. The mode of family therapy for this program has emphasized a flexible approach in working with small groupings or whole families as the issues dictate rather than a rigid insistence on seeing the whole family at every visit.

Prevention of Mental Illness. For many families, one person's treatment is another person's prevention. For example, attention paid to the conflicts or posthospital adjustment of a mother can prevent developmental problems in her child, and development of a good therapeutic relationship with a mother will allow her to discuss her child's problem earlier. Other types of prevention programs include sex education groups, teen discussion groups in the schools, obese adolescent groups at the YMCA, and mental health input into the health education activities of the health center such as childbirth preparation, nutrition, and health education programs.

Psychosomatic Medicine. The conceptual split between mental and physical health care in our country has made integration difficult at the service level. The neighborhood health center is an ideal setting to correct this, with its opportunities for psychiatrist, internist, and nurse to work closely together around illnesses such as peptic ulcer, asthma, and hypertension. However, merely being part of a health center does not bring this kind of close cooperation automatically. There has, at times, been a tendency for some staff to "refer and forget." One method we have had to counteract this has been joint work on a special project. For example, few hypertensive patients were referred to mental health until the staff psychologist formed a group of patients with a nurse from the hypertension program as coleader. The nurse's relationship with her patients resulted in the lowest "no-show" rate for any group therapy in the center and the blood pressures of three out of five patients in the first group fell significantly below the levels on medication alone with a corresponding decrease in symptomatology. This nurse is now working with a psychologist to broaden her hypertension evaluation to include environmental and interpersonal stress and we are planning a multilevel intervention program in conjunction with the medical school department of psychiatry.

The degree to which subspecialized mental health services are offered at the health center and how they fit into the structure has been another area for development. For example, all adult mental health ambulatory therapies have been offered to advantage at the health center, but the drug addiction services have been more appropriately provided at another site as backup with linkages to the health center.

In the area of child mental health services, RCCHC has had to face the following problem: If full-time, fully trained child psychiatric staff are not available for the health center, should all children be referred to the backup child psychiatry department at the community mental health center, or should the part-time staff from the CMHC child department be relied on to provide services at the neighborhood health center? Because these two alternatives in isolation have been less than optimal, we have arrived at a third: to hire full-time mental health professionals who have had some experience in working with children as well as adults to do child screening, work with families and children around milder developmental problems, and serve as referral agents and liaison with the more intensive child services at the CMHC with which a weekly child diagnostic conference is held. In this manner the general health center staff does not have to relate to a large number of different part-time mental health staff who only treat children, or only consult, and who are from another organization. This results in less fragmentation of interstaff cooperation and lines of responsibility.

Interstaff Relationships

In 1970, one of the original mental health objectives was to enhance communication between physical and mental health staff by sharing the same space and promoting information communication in order to achieve more appropriate timely referrals, more skillful handling of emotional problems by other departments, and more understanding of what mental health services can and cannot do.

By 1976 the mental health program succeeded in developing these informal relationships which have produced productive, satisfying joint work around patient care. Working in the same building has aided greatly in this, although not always easy due to a widespread preconception that if space in a building is tight, then mental health services, being "different," should be the first to find space elsewhere. The frequent opportunity to get a "sidewalk consultation" or immediate additional mental health, physical, or social service attention for one's patient (instead of the long wait for a distant clinic appointment), with a chance to talk to the other provider, has been extremely important for all the staff. Thus, simple physical proximity has been a very important factor in improving our coordination and appropriateness of referral.

The productiveness of the relationship with staff in other departments varies; mental health staff often must make special attempts to "reach" some doctors or nurses, despite the fact that all work in the same environment. Joint work on a project or patient important to the other staff member is one of the most effective ways of promoting communication. Lack of communication between mental health and other staff, on the other hand, may result in few or no mental health referrals, referrals too late in the problem or disease process, inappropriate referrals, or lack of understanding of what may constitute mental health treatment. For example, does the physician view certain decisions for mental health treatment as "dumping a patient" — as in the instance of a referral from internal medicine to mental health, evaluation of the problem and then mental health deciding to follow the patient indirectly through the referring doctor's nurse with out continuing indirect consultation? This, in fact, may be the best quality care in this instance because the patient does not need the special skills of the psychiatrist but does need to continue with a particular, very meaningful nursing relationship. Does the nursing supervisor, in turn, see the work of mental health personnel with her nurse as robbing her staff for purposes of "psychiatric nursing" — is this liaison viewed more positively as enhancing a skill the nurse should routinely carry out with patients?

Emphasis on informal communication has, at times, brought neglect of vital, more formal, communication about patient care, such as adequate written referral requests from the other staff or adequate notes in the patient's chart on the evaluation or treatment in process. Feedback to the referring party, both formal and informal, is vitally necessary, lest the notion develop that "you refer to mental health and nothing ever happens". Often feedback to other staff concerning successes with patients was neglected. This fails to provide a balanced view of total efforts, since failures may seem more evident to a frustrated referring staff member who never hears about the positive side.

Interdepartmental role conflict is more prone to occur when the full range of mental health treatment services is provided within the health center rather than limited staff consultation only. These work conflicts more frequently occur with departments whose function and role are closer, such as the social service department. The RCCHC Mental Health and Social Service departments had been separate because they both originated from different programs which merged to form the health center. Political factors had prevented their integration and resulted in a good deal of role overlap and vague coordination which is being corrected with a planned merger into one department.

The employment of mental health staff on at least a three-quarter time basis at the health center has been important. This has enabled other staff to get to know them as people and to develop working relationships with them. Part-time staff find it difficult to identify with the program, are difficult to reach when needed, may see patients they do not know others are seeing, and usually show that they have little understanding of the life and problems of the health center as a whole.

Family Health Care Teams

In 1970 the original team concept at RCCHC was an interdisciplinary group from a work site or catchment area which shared the health care of a group of families and met together regularly to plan, coordinate, and communicate about this care. The expected byproducts of this team were diminution in both status barriers between staff and rigid vertical departmental lines which interfered with inter-disciplinary coordination.

By 1976, although the teams were not a strictly mental health program function, the mental health department played a major role in developing them as a result of its interest in a healthier, more productive staff climate. Historically, the first teams contained 25 staff, which made for cumbersome meetings in which few were given a chance to speak, and which resembled mini "grand rounds," serving more of an educative than a coordinative function. The staff feared giving a family presentation before such a group. The traditional professional departments (vertical structure) were quite strong, and some saw an interdisci-plinary team (horizontal structure) as a threat to their autonomy, a competitor for their time, or peripheral, and did not really support it with their staff mem-bers (evidenced, for example, by ignoring their staff's nonattendance). Some of the health center's leadership vocally supported the team but did not see it as cost effective and did not actively foster it. The team leader's role was difficult to fill since he or she was often a scapegoat for various other problems. No training in team functioning was given, the families discussed were usually multi-problem, and team meetings were often oriented to social or mental health prob-lems to the exclusion of problems of physical health care. In general, the teams seemed to fade from "benign neglect."

This pattern was reversed after a general review of team function in 1972 which revealed those shortcomings. The solution involved forming smaller, more functional teams of 12, including doctors, nurses, health workers, social service, and mental health. An interdisciplinary "team support committee" was organized which convinced the administration that a team training program, developed at the MIT-Sloan School of Management [8], would make them more productive. Although this training helped, the more important input came from the "support committee" which continued as a backup clearinghouse for the problems of these horizontal groups within a vertically structured organization. They served as leadership trainers, wrote guidelines, and generally acted as buffers for friction within the structure.

Since responsibility within the health center is channeled vertically, the teams do not function as true work units, and do not carry a separate and distinct panel of patients. Their function has been rather to provide a weekly interdisciplinary meeting consisting of case presentations, inservice training, and education about community resources. In this role they have been a useful supplement.

Relationship to the Health Center as a System of Health Care

An important principle of this mental health model has been that if mental health was to be more than just an appendix to the health care at RCCHC, it would have to be an integral part of the organism delivering health care. This involves mental health personnel becoming a part of the system not as "psychiatrist for the institution" but as peer staff members contributing skills to the organization as a whole.

The task of getting "inside" the health center system itself was not easy. At times requests to be part of an interdisciplinary planning effort were met with negative responses indicating that general health care staff felt such efforts were intrusive. Gradually, from 1970 to 1976, through our involvement in health center meetings, projects, and committees embracing many concerns, the mental health staff has come to be seen as "part of the family." We have thus been shaped by the needs of the organization as a whole in its approach to patient service, and we, in turn, have shaped the health center, even though it would many times have been the easier course to withdraw and tend to our own "mental health garden."

Keys to arriving at this position inside the organization have been: (1) heeding the larger goals of a comprehensive health care organization and not exclusively the goals of the mental health department; (2) organizationally remaining under a medical director rather than splitting into a parallel department; (3) playing a part in organizational meetings even though they did not have an obvious mental health agenda; (4) forming coalitions with other departments but avoiding polarization; (5) working on joint clinical projects with other departments; (6) recognizing that a position inside the organizational "family" does not confer the status and role bestowed on an outside consultant, who may gain in short-term leverage but does not have the longer term influence resulting from working from within.

Some of the results of this effort have been the formation of family health care teams, encouraging better communication between staff and top management, facilitating staff communication and problem solving at the site and at total staff meetings, and playing a role in bringing in an outside consultant to help with general organizational matters.

Relationship to the Backup Community Mental Health Center

The RCCHC was first operated by a university medical center (Boston University Medical Center), facilitating an early decision to coordinate the Center's mental health services closely with those of the CMHC affiliated with the parent university (the Solomon Carter Fuller Community Mental Health Center) to avoid duplication and fragmentation of service.

During the course of six years, the Fuller CMHC has served as a backup for the RCCHC services in the areas of inpatient, child services, drug abuse, and alcoholism programs. To assist coordination, the RCCHC mental health director became a member of the clinical services coordinating committee of the CMHC. Referrals have moved in both directions, with most of the referrals from the CMHC to the health center consisting of aftercare.

Problems in the relationship have centered around decentralization issues and the attitudes of many in the academic community about services at a neighborhood health center. The health centers in the CMHC catchment area have asked that the CMHC ambulatory mental health services be delivered through the neighborhood health centers by contractual agreement—an arrangement that had resulted in more comprehensive, more accessible care than separate mental health programs. The CMHC, having few ambulatory staff other than psychiatric residents and other trainees, felt that this staff shortage prevented this arrangement and located its staff at the medical center complex. The CMHC area board, however, will set policy and plan further in this area as it assumes more responsibility from the medical school for the CMHC.

A general impression has existed in this and other academic medical institutions that fully trained mental health professionals who choose to do full-time clinical practice for a community organizaiton must, by virtue of their activity and location, be doing less than adequate work. The reasoning goes something like this: since community practice, teaching, or research takes place in low-income communities, a person wanting to practice there must not have had better job offers; hence, he must be an inferior clinician. Hopefully, this impression is being laid to rest as our visibility increases in the CMHC with which we work, through presentation of our programs and limited teaching involvement in the medical school. Conflicts between staff "insiders" (in the CMHC central unit) and staff "outsiders" (in the neighborhood) can be very damaging to good patient care. Since this relationship has improved we have received more credibility in and access to the CMHC subspecialty services and inpatient units.

The issues of teaching students and residents by having them work at RCCHC has been a difficult one. An initial impetus for the development of the health center was the wish of the community to have access to care other than by the rotating students and residents from the local medical schools. On the other hand, the area board has recognized the need for the introduction and sensitization of students to a neighborhood health center practice so that doctors can be recruited in the future. One possible resolution of this dilemma is the limited and appropriately controlled introduction of students to the health center which will not change the primary responsibility of the full-time health center staff for their patients.

Discussion

In summary, our experience indicates that the neighborhood comprehensive health center is an ideal setting through which to deliver mental health services because "that's where the families are." The tremendous drawing power of such a center has brought us into very close contact with families, providing opportunities for prevention, earlier intervention, and more accessible direct services. The Center itself has shaped the mental health service within it to the needs of a neighborhood and to the comprehensive health program itself. Our experience with this Center has been reviewed in this chapter in the areas of patient accessibility, range of mental health services, interstaff relationship to the health center as a system of health care, and relationship to the backup CMHC.

A variety of primary care and comprehensive health programs have arisen based on various funding structures—OEO, HEW, MIC, HMO, municipal, third-party payments, and so forth. Although each of these has its special problems and needs, most of the more general findings outlined in this chapter can apply whether programs are in poor or affluent communities. In short, we advocate a strong mental health service operating within comprehensive health programs with full or majority-time mental health staff identified with the program working in side-by-side physical proximity with the health center staff, decentralized into the health teams of the program, offering a full spectrum of mental health services, and playing significant roles in the life of the comprehensive health program itself.

A comprehensive program functioning in accord with the above characteristics has a number of inherent advantages over separate health and mental health delivery programs; the advantages include:

1. The family orientation of mental health services is enhanced by virtue of practicing in a program which must respond to the total health needs of a family.

2. Increased accessibility and acceptability of mental health services to patients results from a combination of factors, such as the decreased stigma attached to mental health services when they are part of a general health care program rather than separate, and less patient resistance to referral within an organization than to referral between organizations [9].

3. Increased coordination of care results from increased knowledge about and informal communication between mental health and other health care providers.

4. Opportunities for primary and secondary prevention are increased due to the greater access to the milestones and crises of family life, enhancing the development of special programs for higher-risk groups (i.e., waiting-room child development education, prenatal groups, and so forth).

5. Psychosomatic illness is more effectively treated in an integrated setting and decreases inappropriate utilization of medical services. Since early signs of maladaptive responses to life stresses may be somatic, the patient often turns first to a trusted physician or nurse. If mental health services are closely linked to this health care, they may directly or indirectly have beneficial impact in this early stage of problem formation.

6. Manpower efficiency is enhanced by such joint programs, which results in decreased duplication of personal counseling, provides health care staff with more available consultation to improve their skills in the psychological aspect of their health care delivery, and may reduce utilization of medical services [10,11].

7. The mental health staff may be of help to the entire health program in areas of improving its approach to consumers, provider interrelationships, and psychological aspects of patient care management.

A word about funding is necessary as the funding source is crucial in determining what shape a program will take. For example, a shortage of funds for mental health services in poor areas has resulted in "consultation only" programs. Complete dependence on a hodgepodge of categorical grants has resulted in misshappen, out-of-balance programs which must enter into frantic game-playing situations with their many funding sources to stay alive. The only forces shaping the program should in fact be the needs of the patients and the resources to provide services, rather than a series of special categorical sources.

The central question seems to be: As federal monies are now being distributed to the states, what share will be provided for mental health services through comprehensive health programs? Who will be their advocate?—the state departments of mental health, or are they too wedded to maintaining their separate mental health institutions and structures? The community mental health centers, or are they too committed to their separate clinics and fears of a general health "takeover"? The city or state public health departments, or are they too preoccupied with hospitals, categorical clinics, and not offending the solo practitioners? The staffs of the Comprehensive Programs, or are they too separate and divided? The comprehensive health program boards, or are they too preoccupied with providing physical health care only and will simply accept the split between mental health care and primary health care that has been handed to them by the professionals? A logical coalition for the development of more mental health services within comprehensive health programs is one composed of consumers, enlightened health planners on the federal and state level who can write guidelines recognizing the advantages of these integrated programs, and community mental health centers who can see the advantages of locating their services in a comprehensive health program.

What should be the relationship between these community mental health centers (CMHCs) and neighborhood health centers (NHCs)? At least four types of relationships are possible: (1) the NHC patients needing mental health services are sent to the separate CMHC; (2) a pseudopod of the CMHC extends into the NHC; (3) part of the CMHC funds or staff are allocated to the NHC to be used to deliver the mental health services for that neighborhood through the NHC, linked to a CMHC network; (4) the NHC receives separate mental health funding from whatever source (capitation, state grant, third party) to deliver its mental health program and then associates itself with the local CMHC to ensure coordination of service. In our experience only through the last two models will a mental health service emerge that can effectively utilize all that a comprehensive neighborhood health center has to offer for better mental health service to the consumer.

References

1. Goldensohn, S.S., Fink, R., and Shapiro, S. Referral, Utilization, and Staffing Patterns of a Mental Health Service in a Prepaid Group Practice Program in New York. *Am. J. Psychiat.* 126, 135-143, 1969.

2. Goldensohn, S.S. A Prepaid Group Practice Mental Health Service as Part of a Health Maintenance Organization. *Am. J. Orthopsychiat.* 42, 154-158, 1972.

3. Gibson, R.W. Can Mental Health Be Included in the Health Maintenance Organization? *Am. J. Psychiat.* 128, 33-40, 1972.

4. Morrill, R.G. A New Mental Health Services Model for the Comprehensive Neighborhood Health Center. *Am. J. Pub. Health.* 62, 1108-1111, 1972.

5. _____. Health Center Setting Cited as Best for Patients, Psychiatrists. Roche Report, *Frontiers of Psychiatry*, 3, 1-11, 1973.

6. _____. Comprehensive Mental Health through a Neighborhood Health Center in *Mental Health, the Public Health Challenge*, ed., Lieberman, E.J., *Am. Pub. Health Assn.*, 1975. p. 120-124.

7. Borus, J.F., Janowitch, L.A., Kieffer, F., Morrill, R.G., Reich, L., Simone, E., Towle, L. The Coordination of Mental Health Services at the Neighborhood Level. *Am. J. Psychiat.* 132, 11, 1975. p. 1177-1181.

8. Wise, H., Beckhard, R., Rubin, E., and Kyte, A. *Making Health Teams Work.* Ballinger, 1974. Cambridge, Mass.

9. Fink, R., Shapiro, S., Goldensohn, S.S., and Daily, E.F. The "Filter-Down" Process to Psychiatry in a Group Practice Medical Care Program. *Am. J. Pub. Health.* 59, 245-260, 1969.

10. Follette, W., and Cummings, N.A. Psychiatric Services and Medical Utilization in a Prepaid Health Plan Setting. *Medical Care.* 5, 25-35, 1967.

11. Goldberg, I.D., Krantz, G., and Locke, B.Z. Effect of a Short-Term Out-Patient Psychiatric Therapy Benefit on the Prepaid Group Practice Medical Program. *Medical Care.* 8, 419-428, 1970.

9

An Outreach Team Approach to Neighborhood Mental Health Services

Martin M. Norman

Despite the important trend toward more comprehensive care at the neighborhood level, delivery of vital human services to low-income, urban consumers is generally fragmented and disorganized. As a result, many high-risk community residents remain either outside the existing network of human services or else hopelessly entangled within it, unwilling or unable to make adequate use of the care so often desperately needed. On the other hand, the absence of coordinated systems of client care often results in duplication of effort and a waste of scarce community resources. Opportunities for early case finding are frequently sacrificed to the need for crisis intervention. In this regard, many small, well-established community agencies, with unique opportunities to facilitate preventative interventions, remain outside the mainstream of traditional mental health support. Inadequate information about utilization of existing neighborhood resources is as serious a problem as the absence of critical resources.

This chapter describes a model of neighborhood mental health outreach developed within a primarily low-income urban community. The outreach model evolved in response to service delivery problems at different neighborhood levels. First, whether due to limited resources or rigid institutional policies, systematic outreach and advocacy services to consumers have not been an integral component of neighborhood health care services provided by hospitals and health centers. Second, similar restrictions have also limited the range, scope, and intensity of consultative outreach services to community agencies. As a result, cross-referral linkages between neighborhood agencies and surrounding health centers and hospitals are often formal, impersonal, and underutilized. Finally, the dearth of collaborative neighborhood-wide mechanisms for information sharing and program planning has been a serious impediment to the development of comprehensive strategies of service intervention and coordination.

Design and Structure of the Outreach Model

The outreach model of neighborhood intervention described here is derived from

The author wishes to thank Rebekah Norman and the staff of the Jamaica Plain Outreach Program for their assistance, support, and dedication in the preparation of this chapter and program participation.

the experiences of the Jamaica Plain Community Mental Health Outreach Program (JPOP) in Boston, Massachusetts. This program is funded in large part by a National Institute of Mental Health (NIMH) staffing grant and is affiliated with the Massachusetts Mental Health Center, a community mental health center, and the Judge Baker Guidance Center, a private, nonprofit child guidance center, both also located in Boston.

Goals of the Model

The outreach program has three primary goals. The first involves the development of a broad, grass-roots referral network geared to identifying and engaging high-risk individuals and families on an early intervention basis; accessibility and flexibility of services is an essential dimension of such a goal.

The second central objective is to maximize the quality of mental health care by coordinating the existing human services network in a neighborhood. This necessitates a thorough and personalized familiarity with the target neighborhood.

The third goal of the outreach model is to identify critical problems and gaps in service delivery and then to facilitate neighborhood-wide approaches aimed at addressing such concerns through social advocacy and/or collaborative program planning efforts.

Characteristics of the Model

A pivotal criterion of the outreach model is the need for a flexible and mobile orientation to service delivery in a neighborhood. Therefore, instead of working from a single neighborhood base, the central characteristic of the outreach model is the formation of a grass roots network of multiple neighborhood bases. Because the central consideration is reaching people in distress, the setting for service delivery must be as accessible as possible. For that reason a majority of the direct service visits are provided to clients within their own homes. In addition, a range of alternative neighborhood sites are used to provide direct services. Together these multiple sites of convenient service delivery serve to underscore the free-floating orientation of the outreach approach.

A second characteristic of the outreach model involves the degree and intensity of collaborative relationships fostered between outreach staff and neighborhood providers. Professional interactions are rarely limited to regularly scheduled meetings. Rather, such a format is a foundation upon which reciprocal, informal calls or visits occur as needs arise. Accessibility to neighborhood providers is as essential an outreach feature as is accessibility to consumers. Personalized working relationships between outreach and neighborhood providers are

heightened by frequent, multilevel interactions, ranging from direct service collaborations to joint participation on neighborhood committees concerned with
social advocacy.

A third characteristic of the model involves the nature of neighborhood
affiliations. The outreach approach attempts to identify and deal with the
neighborhood as a total system rather than with any one part of it. In order to
play a network-spanning role, it is essential that the primary affiliations of the
outreach team be with mental health institutions outside the neighborhood.
Programmatic flexibility to respond to neighborhood-wide priorities for service
delivery is maximized when there is no financial dependence on any one neighborhood agency.

Characteristics of the Target Neighborhood

Jamaica Plain, a section of Boston, is a neighborhood of contrasts. Densely
populated, approximately 45,000 people live within an area of 5 square miles.
These boundaries contain, at one end of the economic spectrum, affluent sections
consisting of very fashionable one- and two-family homes; residents in this section of the neighborhood generally have a high educational, occupational and
income status. At the other end of the spectrum there are housing projects in
which a growing number of families, primarily black and Spanish-surname, are
living at or near the poverty level. Between these two poles, the majority of
community residents consist of white, second and third generation, working-
class Irish Catholic families. However, the neighborhood is very much in transition, and Jamaica Plain increasingly has become a racially and economically
diverse melting pot. As part of Boston, it finds itself struggling to cope with
most of the major stresses of urban life, accentuated by the additional pressure
of a federal school desegregation order. With a long and proud political history
behind it, Jamaica Plain is alive and teeming with a strong and articulate network
of community action committees and groups. While often duplicating efforts
and frequently at odds with one another, these committees are broadly representative of the different constituencies served and generally effective in bringing about community change.

Service Gaps and Target Groups

There are three neighborhood health centers in Jamaica Plain and mental health
services are available at all of them. However, due in large part to financial
limitations, mental health staff are primarily part-time and are provided through
affiliations with backup teaching hospitals. The combination of heavy service
demands and limited time leave little opportunity for the more time-consuming

efforts needed to reach out to less motivated clients. In addition, the majority of available mental health services are for adults. Significant gaps in service thus result for three primary target groups: children and youth, the elderly, and the Spanish-speaking.

The children and youth, most at risk, are usually the least willing to utilize traditional community agencies for supportive services. Rather, they rely on more familiar drop-in centers and other social hangouts. With few exceptions, these locales are without any systematic mental health support or contact. Despite increasing rates of school truancy and dropout, minimal efforts at service coordination have existed between the public schools and the rest of the network of human services in the neighborhood. The result is an absence of any early screening or preventive intervention strategies.

The second critical service gap involves the elderly. Jamaica Plain has one of the largest and growing elderly populations in the city. A total of thirty nursing homes operates in the neighborhood. The single most pressing and unmet problem in this area is the large number of isolated and impoverished elderly, by and large untouched by the wealth of available community services. Hospitals and health centers have not committed the necessary outreach resources needed to seek out and try to draw these high-risk senior citizens into the health care network. At the same time, consultation supports provided by community mental health agencies are limited and fragmented. A clear lack of any neighborhood-wide focus on service collaboration and advocacy planning for the elderly has thus persisted.

The third area of significant service need has involved the large number of Hispanic residents in Jamaica Plain. Over a period of five years, the Spanish population in the area has nearly doubled, comprising approximately 20 percent of the neighborhood and making it the single largest minority group. Jamaica Plain, as well as the city of Boston as a whole, has few Hispanic providers, both professional and nonprofessional. Jamaica Plain has a single, small Spanish center run by a local poverty agency, offering only limited employment counseling and interpreter services. The small number of Hispanic mental health providers work primarily at hospitals or health centers and have little or no time to reach out to high-risk families or consult with community agencies. Most striking are the scattered efforts at resource planning and service coordination in light of the critical need to expand services to Spanish residents of all ages.

Linkages

The keystone of the outreach model is the pattern and quality of linkages established between the outreach staff and (1) the backup hospitals and mental health centers, (2) the neighborhood health centers, and (3) selected human service agencies and institutions serving the neighborhood.

Backup Hospitals and Mental Health Centers

The JPOP is supported primarily by a community mental health staffing grant funded by the NIMH. Additional administrative and limited financial support is provided by the two Harvard-affiliated backup institutions to the JPOP: Massachusetts Mental Health Center (MMHC) and the Judge Baker Guidance Center (JBGC). MMHC is a comprehensive community mental health center serving a catchment area of over 200,000 residents. Jamaica Plain is one of five geographic neighborhoods within that catchment area. While mental health services are available to people of all ages, the inpatient facilities have been primarily oriented toward older adolescents and adults. JBGC is a private, nonprofit child guidance center without any set geographic boundaries for service delivery. It offers a full range of individual and family treatment approaches with particular emphasis on intensive, long-term psychotherapy. In addition, it houses a day school for children with learning problems. Finally, in affiliation with Children's Hospital Medical Center, the JBGC has inpatient facilities for children with psychosomatic problems.

In developing and sponsoring the JPOP, both institutions agreed to provide, on a priority basis, extended diagnostic and treatment care to clients referred by the outreach staff. In turn, the JPOP receives direct referrals from the backup centers when it is determined that Jamaica Plain clients are considered unlikely or unable to sustain regular hospital appointments. For purposes of coordination, designated staff members from the JPOP serve as liaison to each of the two institutions. These linkages serve multiple purposes. The emphasis on personal lines of communication facilitates reciprocal intake and referral procedures. In addition, personal linkages increase the opportunities for mutual consultation and education, as such interchange occurs around case conference and individual client consultations. In addition, the outreach staff present their approaches to neighborhood intervention periodically as part of the sequence of formal conferences/rounds at the backup centers. Finally, JPOP administrative staff attend community resource and program planning meetings with administrative staff at the backup centers.

Neighborhood Health Centers

Within the neighborhood itself, the three comprehensive health centers are pivotal resources. In order for the outreach approach to extend services beyond these existing resources, it is essential that collaborative ties to the health network be solid. Even more than with the affiliated backup hospitals, the JPOP model necessitates a reciprocal resource relationship with the neighborhood health centers. The outreach program encourages the use of neighborhood health centers whenever possible. However, because many residents, for whatever reasons, are uncomfortable or unwilling to use the neighborhood facilities, it is important that the outreach program be identified by the neighborhood as autonomous from the health centers.

JPOP linkages to the neighborhood health centers, like those to the backup hospitals, are focused in the areas of case referral, coordination, consultation, and administrative planning and review. A member of the JPOP staff is assigned as principal liaison to each of the three health centers. This entails establishing personal and regular contacts with health center staff responsible for intake and referral. At these meetings cases referred to the JPOP are brought by the staff liaison to weekly outreach intake meetings. Similarly, cases to be referred to the neighborhood health center are discussed at health center intake meetings. The mutual understanding is that cases will be accepted on a priority basis. In addition, JPOP staff periodically participate in case review meetings with the health center's medical or mental health teams. Administratively, the health center directors provide the JPOP staff with limited office space that can be used for both client and staff meetings. In addition, one health center is designated as the central storage facility for the confidential records of the JPOP. The JPOP director meets periodically with the health center directors to review staff collaboration and to participate in neighborhood-wide health planning meetings.

Neighborhood Agencies and Institutions

Building on a base of affiliations and linkages with the backup hospitals and the neighborhood health centers, the essence of the outreach approach is the establishment of close working ties with the other human service providers in the neighborhood. Because of the free-floating orientation of the outreach team, such linkages include multiple outreach service sites based in selected neighborhood agencies and institutions. A general consideration for outreach site selection is the necessity that locations be geographically distributed across the entire neighborhood. A specific consideration is the need to ensure that outreach sites are spread among the range of agencies, regardless of size, which provide the critical human services for the target population. In many neighborhoods, the smaller agencies establish the strongest credibility because of the informal and personal style of their staff. Frequently, many neighborhood residents will turn first to such agencies in a time of crisis.

The JPOP has focused its linkages to neighborhood-wide agencies in three areas: welfare, the schools, and the police. One or more of these systems play a significant role in the lives of practically all of the clients served by the outreach team. The entry process in each of the three agencies included extensive administrative planning meetings that focused on service needs and goals and the nature of possible staff collaborations. In these discussions, the central factor which enhanced the development of linkages was the JPOP's stated goals of on-site direct service as well as facilitating neighborhood-wide networks of service coordination. With respect to the local office of the Welfare Department, the JPOP assigned a staff member as principal liaison to meet regularly with welfare workers in three designated areas: Care and Protection, Intake and Referral, and Assistance Payment. In the public schools, outreach liaison staff were assigned to a total of nine schools, from elementary to high school, serving the neighborhood [3] . Finally, principal contact with the police was established through the District Police Station located in the neighborhood. An outreach staff member met informally at the police station with the juvenile probation officer and other police officers. Other linkages in areas related to legal matters included on-site case referral and collaboration with the staff of the neighborhood legal aid office and with the manager and staff of the Neighborhood City Hall, a local branch of Central City Hall in Boston. While the most formal and extensively used outreach service sites were established in the schools, outreach staff were also provided space for client interviews on an "as needed" basis at the other contact sites.

The process of developing alliances with smaller neighborhood agencies was considerably more informal. In the area of children and youth, attention focused on several of the small after-school and evening drop-in centers. Frequent outreach staff meetings with both center directors and their staff provided the groundwork for developing rapport and accessibility. Furthermore, because the group of children and youth using particular centers remain fairly constant, recognition and familiarity of outreach staff was enhanced with target individuals. Contact with drop-in centers frequently had a ripple effect in that it often led to contacts with other neighborhood youth street-work programs.

For younger children, the JPOP established collaborative links with a neighborhood-wide preschool program and several day care programs. These programs provided the JPOP on-site space for child and parent interviews.

With regard to services for the elderly, a principal linkage of the JPOP was with a large neighborhood housing project for the elderly. After planning with the project manager, an outreach staff member specializing in geriatrics established an outreach service delivery base in the project. Other direct outreach bases were established at each of the three small senior drop-in centers located across the neighborhood.

Finally, in addition to the network of formal linkages throughout the neighborhood, JPOP staff fostered informal ties with some of the neighborhood's most respected and utilized "informal" providers whenever possible—the variety and drug store operators. Owned by local residents with long-standing reputations for providing help in a crisis, these storekeepers welcomed the opportunity for support and referral offered by the JPOP.

Staffing Pattern and JPOP Structure

The staffing pattern of the JPOP was designed to match its mission of reaching and serving the principal target groups to whom neighborhood mental health services were to be directed. Specifically, each staff member was selected for expertise with one of the three target groups. For children and youth, there is a full-time child psychologist (who also serves as Program Director), a full-time psychiatric social worker, and part-time child psychiatrist. In the area of services to the Spanish-speaking, the staff includes a full-time bilingual psychiatric social worker and a half-time native Hispanic psychologist. Finally, with regard to the elderly, a full-time geriatric social worker and a full-time, noncredentialed community mental health coordinator provide services. The latter staff member is a resident of the local community and has extensive experience working with senior citizens. A second full-time, noncredentialed community mental health coordinator, also a community resident, provides a combination of outreach counseling, case advocacy, and neighborhood resource coordination skills in conjunction with staff in each of the three target group areas. In addition to the program director, administrative work is carried out by an administrative assistant who is a neighborhood resident. The assistant is responsible for staff scheduling coordination, development of record and bill-keeping systems, and overall communication management at the outreach storefront. Regular staff supervision is provided by the program director as well as by a senior social worker on the staff of the Massachusetts Mental Health Center based full time in Jamaica Plain.

The entire outreach team has two regularly scheduled meetings each week: a general staff meeting and a case intake and review meeting, both held in the outreach storefront. During the general staff meeting, there is time for informal exchange of neighborhood and client information as well as for program planning. Because collaboration with neighborhood agencies is such an extensive and critical aspect of the outreach team's work, the progress and problems encountered by the outreach staff in this area are reviewed periodically with the aid of an agency collaboration index file. Each index card contains information regarding each agency, including the names and roles of the key liaison staff and the frequency and nature of outreach contact. Finally, general staff meetings are used as times to invite other neighborhood providers to discuss and review ongoing collaborative ties.

The case intake and review meetings specifically focus on clinical issues. New referrals are discussed and ongoing cases are reviewed briefly or more extensively, depending on need. In order to ensure continuity of client care, follow-up on outreach cases is essential. Toward this end the JPOP developed a card file index that results in automatic periodic review of every ongoing case. When a case is opened, a date for review is noted on the case index file, and each time the case is brought up, a new date is listed until the time the case is considered closed.

With the exception of these two planned meetings, the remainder of the outreach team's time is spent elsewhere in the neighborhood. Daily staff schedules are posted in the storefront so that staff can be reached when needed.

Agency Collaborations

Within the framework of the outreach model, agency collaboration refers broadly to a set of multilevel work relationships between members of the outreach staff and members of one or more neighborhood agency staffs. Such levels of collaboration include a focus on service delivery within an individual agency, interagency coordination of services, and systems intervention.

Collaborations with Individual Agencies

While the type of outreach services provided to each neighborhood agency varies with the specific needs of different settings, a basic common denominator is the personalized orientation of outreach staff. Combining regularly scheduled meetings with periodic informal visits and/or phone contact, outreach staff emphasize their responsiveness. Organizationally, outreach staff are individually assigned to neighborhood agencies based as much as possible on their interest and expertise. Initial efforts at each agency are focused on providing support at whatever level the agency feels help is most needed. As collaborative relationships evolve, and outreach staff become known and trusted, exploration of an agency's needs may broaden from a crisis focus to issues of long-range planning and staff development

A small, well-established neighborhood settlement house serving children and youth was forced to limit services due to shrinking financial support. Lack of resources prevented the settlement house from being able to reach out to parents of the children served. Despite a clear need for staff education and consultation, the request for help focused on direct services to families whose children appeared to be in crisis. Intervening at the crisis level first, the outreach worker was later able to use the work accomplished with families as the basis for a more generalized series of staff discussions. Over a period of time, the collaborative relationship grew to the point where the staff felt comfortable in requesting that the outreach worker serve as a resource to the staff in assisting them to review and plan programmatic directions for the center.

In this example, the combination of direct services, informal case consultations, and program consultations were provided primarily by the assigned outreach worker with additional client intervention support from the other members of the outreach team. The flexibility of the outreach worker to comfortably shift to different levels of agency need proved to enhance greatly the overall effectiveness of intervention.

Another example involving services for the elderly illustrates the multiplier effect the outreach team often had.

A member of the JPOP was assigned to a newly opened senior housing project that served approximately 300 elders. Administrated by a part-time manager, the project was without any social services. The outreach worker's initial focus, after establishing an informal consultative relationship, was on providing direct services for seniors in the project. This involved regular visits to their apartments, where counseling support was offered. At the same time, ongoing discussions with the manager regarding service needs and available community resources led to the development of a small social service team based in the project, composed of staff from several other community agencies dealing with senior citizens. The outreach worker then was able to shift the primary focus of outreach attention from direct services to program consultation and resource coordination.

Interagency Coordination of Services

Insufficient communication and planning among human service providers results in a waste of already limited agency resources in a neighborhood. Opportunities to assist in the development of comprehensive and coordinated approaches to client care are among the most valuable aspects of the outreach model. Combining a familiarity with neighborhood resources and personal contacts with many key agency providers, outreach staff are in a unique position to facilitate convening representatives of service networks for purposes of resource coordination, program planning, and systematic management of individual client care.

A special services coordinator in a public school had frequent need to refer children to the neighborhood health centers for medical and psychiatric services. In trying to do so, she repeatedly encountered difficulties establishing direct lines of communication with central intake personnel at each of the three health centers. School personnel needed to have clear knowledge of health center procedures, service capacity and availability, and information and record-sharing policies. In order to facilitate interagency linkages, a JPOP staff member based at the school as a resource consultant convened a meeting of the relevant personnel from the school and the three health centers.

The area most sorely needing coordination of interagency services is that involving direct client care. In their role as resource liaisons to neighborhood agencies, outreach staff are frequently referred clients known by the referring agency to be involved with other neighborhood agencies. Prior to accepting the referral, the outreach liaison offers consultation support to the referring providers in order to help them pull together existing services and then determine whether additional help is needed. In many instances, contact between providers such as street workers and welfare workers may not have been made because of mutual distrust and/or stereotyped attitudes. In other instances, providers are often unaware of both the role and the participation of other providers. With the outreach workers functioning as catalysts, interagency meetings are convened in order to clarify the roles and goals of participating providers. The outreach staff work to keep the focus on the common goal of all, the well being of the client, a focus often lost in the confusion.

A worker in a neighborhood health center wished to refer a Spanish teenage boy to the JPOP for counseling. Upon inquiry by the outreach liaison to the health center, it was learned that the father was being treated at a community mental health center, the mother was receiving counseling from a neighborhood Spanish agency, another child had been referred to the health center for medical and psychological evaluation, and a welfare worker was actively involved with the family and seeking recreational resources for another child. Working with the agency provider and with the permission of a grateful but thoroughly overwhelmed family, the outreach worker helped arrange a conference of all providers. As a result of this meeting, an agreement was reached to coordinate services through a single prime agency which would take the responsibility for scheduling periodic joint review meetings.

The broader intent of the JPOP's coordination efforts is to provide a model for neighborhood agencies which will lead to future "multiplier" effects in serving other clients as well.

Systems Intervention

Drawing upon diversified knowledge accumulated through repeated experiences coordinating human service networks, and serving both agencies and consumers, outreach staff are in a central position to identify neighborhood-wide gaps in information-sharing and service delivery. An important extension of the outreach model is the need to use such knowledge in the service of helping to bring about broader system change in the neighborhood.

In each of its target areas, JPOP staff takes an active role in participating in both neighborhood planning councils and catchment-area-wide human services committees. Joining with colleagues from surrounding neighborhoods, an important aim of JPOP staff is to encourage the development of centralized information and referral systems, together with production of new or updated directories of community resources. Thus, where viable community advocacy councils already existed, JPOP staff worked to support and assist these councils. However, where there was a need to develop advocacy boards for specific target groups, JPOP staff took an active role in the organizing process. This function was greatly facilitated by the multiple collaborative relationships developed by outreach staff throughout the neighborhood.

Services to adolescents in the neighborhood were both fragmented and limited. Working together with other key teen providers, JPOP staff helped establish a youth advocacy board. Broadly representative, and with a JPOP staff member serving as co-chairperson, the youth advocacy board was initially formed in order to coordinate information regarding teen services and to identify critical areas of service need. The board, in time, also became a forum for neighborhood discussion of such teen problems as street crime and alcoholism. Now legally incorporated, the board is planning to develop proposals for neighborhood-wide teen programs.

In sum, working simultaneously on different but interrelated levels of agency collaboration, the outreach model aims to effect both short-term change for neighborhood agencies and the consumers they serve, and long-term change in the system of human services delivery for the neighborhood.

Direct Services for Clients

Client referrals to the JPOP come from a wide range of neighborhood agencies and institutions. This is a direct outgrowth of the collaborative relationships developed between outreach staff and neighborhood providers at multiple agency sites. At various neighborhood outreach bases, JPOP staff liaisons meet regularly with agency providers in order to discuss ways to identify and refer clients in distress as early as possible. Because the common characteristic of clients referred is the client's inability and/or refusal to seek needed support from the existing system of neighborhood human services, the strategies of outreach intervention vary, depending on the referral source and the nature of the request for help.

Outreach Counseling

The majority of the low-income, high-risk individuals and families served by the JPOP live from one crisis to another; the crises are physical and financial as well as emotional. Crisis situations that have demanded immediate attention by JPOP workers have included suicide attempts, child abuse, and problems stemming from severe alcoholism. At the same time, for example, families have turned to outreach staff when faced with housing evictions and cutbacks in food stamps. In order to maintain the flexibility and availability to respond to crises, as well as to serve large numbers of clients, the focus of direct counseling is on short-term interventions. These are flexibly defined to allow for meetings ranging from a few weeks to several months. In some instances, outreach staff provide extended care to those clients at risk who are considered to be unable to accept long-term care as provided at community mental health centers.

For a majority of clients referred to the JPOP, initial visits are held in their homes. Otherwise, meetings are held at an accessible outreach site. Appointment times are geared to be as accommodating as possible.

In the area of children and youth, the two most recurrent types of presenting problems involve severe learning and behavior problems in school and delinquent activities around the neighborhood. In school-related problems [3], young children are generally interviewed in school but meetings are also held in their home or in office space provided at a convenient neighborhood agency. Parent interviews are held at home and/or at school. With parental permission, outreach workers work closely with school personnel throughout the intervention process.

A 10-year-old boy was consistently truant from school. The family pattern was chaotic: the parents were separated, although living in the same neighborhood; the father was alcoholic and abusive and the mother had severe emotional problems that prevented her from giving consistent support to the child. At the conclusion of the outreach evaluation, the outreach social worker offered to meet with the mother at home for an extended series of visits. These meetings focused on issues of child and home management, as well as helping the mother seek out needed long-term psychiatric care for herself. With regard to the child, the outreach team psychologist began a series of informal meetings focused on helping the child return to school as well as to better understand and deal with the problems at home. Meeting at first in a local neighborhood agency, they agreed upon a checklist system of recording days of school attended or missed. At the periodic conclusion of a specific number of school days attended, the two of them would take reward trips around the city. This particular approach allowed the child, who had otherwise refused to talk to counselors, not only to return to school, which he did, but also provided him the opportunity to develop a therapeutic relationship comfortably.

Outreach to adolescents requires the greatest flexibility. Initial visits may occur in a school, but are apt to be more effective in a neighborhood locale such as a drop-in center or variety store hangout. Such sites offer the further advantage of teaming up an outreach worker with an agency provider with whom a teen already has a trusting relationship.

An adolescent boy, chronically truant from school and suspected of delinquent activities, was referred to a JPOP worker by a guidance counselor in his high school and by a juvenile probation officer. He refused the recommendation of both to seek help. Informed of this, the outreach worker began to visit a teen drop-in center where the youth frequently hung around. Introduced warmly by the teen center director, the outreach worker and the youth got acquainted over a game of pool. The adolescent found it hard to believe the worker could be the same person he was supposed to get in touch with for help. After several days of pool games, the youth agreed to meet informally with the outreach worker and the teen director in the latter's home in order to discuss the youth's admitted concerns.

The most pressing problem with regard to the elderly involves reaching socially isolated seniors. Most often living alone, these seniors are confronted with multiple problems relating to loss of health, friends, and finances. The process of outreach to such clients is a slow one marked by persistent and frequent home visits. Once access is gained and an assessment of needs is made, the outreach focus widens to helping the seniors take advantage of available neighborhood resources. Combining counseling as well as transportation to resources, the outreach worker helps isolated seniors gradually move outside their homes. If this fails, outreach efforts are instead directed at providing continuing care to the senior at home.

A 65-year-old woman who repeatedly did not follow-up on social service and medical care appointments at neighborhood agencies and health centers was hospitalized at a community mental health center for severe emotional problems related to chronic alcoholism. Upon release from the hospital, she was referred to the JPOP for neighborhood-based follow-up care. Beginning with a few hospital visits prior to release, the outreach worker met with the woman at her home on a frequent basis. The outreach focus was on the client's alcohol problems as well as on multiple problems in living, including financial and medical needs. Over a period of time, the worker assisted the client in keeping medical appointments as well as joining a local church society for serving social and religious needs. The worker also helped secure increased financial benefits from Social Security.

Case Advocacy

As part of a broader counseling involvement with clients, outreach workers frequently find it essential to take on the role of case advocate. This usually entails assisting clients in their efforts to obtain needed goods and services from community institutions. Intimidated and confused by bureaucratic procedures and red tape, many clients fail to take advantage of, or even know about, many services to which they are entitled. An important asset of the outreach staff is their personal familiarity with providers and knowledge of supportive services available within various community institutions. Such contacts and information have frequently facilitated the case advocacy process.

An 80-year-old woman experiencing problems of emotional confusion and time and place disorientation was referred to the JPOP by a community mental health center. Threatened with eviction because of her inability to keep track of rent payments, the woman was terrified that she would be placed in a nursing home. A home assessment by the outreach worker indicated that the woman also had serious difficulties in the areas of personal hygiene as well as general upkeep of her apartment. The principal focus for outreach intervention involved developing a series of protective and supportive services for the woman. Working with a lawyer from a legal aid society, the outreach worker arranged for a conservatorship to help the woman manager her money and keep her apartment. In addition, the worker arranged for the provision of both a visiting nurse and a homemaker service. Finally, the woman was enrolled in a daily meals-on-wheels program run by a local senior drop-in center.

Resource Referral and Liaison

Helping consumers learn about and use the neighborhood resources is a further direct service provided by outreach staff. Many of the clients served by the JPOP staff are in need of a wide range of supportive services. When outreach workers refer clients to neighborhood resources, it is important to see that the recommended services are made available — and with a minimum of confusion and red tape. For this reason, outreach staff serve frequently as resource liaisons. At times such support may simply involve a phone call establishing a personal contact for a client to be seen in an agency or institution. However, for confused and overwhelmed clients, it may be necessary for the outreach worker to provide direct transportation in order to insure that a client gets to an agency appointment on time. In some cases, this may also require assisting a client through an intake or application process at such institutions as hospitals or the Welfare Department.

Finally, because of the link with backup hospitals, outreach staff have also been available to serve in reverse fashion as neighborhood liaisons in cases of crisis for hospital clients from the neighborhood.

A 14-year-old Spanish girl, hospitalized for a suicide attempt, left the hospital without the permission or knowledge of the hospital psychiatrist treating her. Because of the risk the girl presented to herself, the JPOP was consulted and requested to assist in finding and trying to encourage the girl to return for further help. A Spanish outreach worker located the girl at her home and had an extended discussion with her regarding the need to return to the hospital for further psychiatric help. Although ambivalent about doing so, the girl phoned the hospital and agreed to come in for an appointment.

The Outreach Model and the Existing Health Service System: Discussion

Over the last decade or so, the growth and expansion of both community mental health centers (CMHCs) and neighborhood health centers (NHCs) have increased the accessibility and utilization of primary health and mental health services significantly. Nevertheless, many low-income people remain outside the health care system. In order to reach these people, mental health outreach services need to be included as an integral component of the service program at both community mental health and neighborhood health centers [4]. For differing but interrelated reasons, this has generally not yet happened.

One major obstacle for community mental health centers has been the repeated cutbacks in funding and resulting shortages of staff. Providing community-based care to populations as large as 200,000, the staff of a community mental health center are continually faced with service demands that exceed the supply of available manpower. The development of outreach and advocacy services requires the presence of staff with the flexibility and mobility to spend significant periods in the neighborhood establishing a personal familiarity with the many grass-roots agencies that comprise the total human services network. In times of financial shortage, maintenance of vital hospital or center-based services tends to take priority over neighborhood-based services.

Another significant obstacle has been the limited scope of training that mental health professionals receive in the area of understanding and dealing with the multiple problems of the disadvantaged. In many mental health centers, training models focus primarily on the intrapsychic and interpersonal dynamics of the individual. The conceptual framework is not sufficiently broadened to include the impact the overall psychosocial matrix has on the lives of low-income and minority clients. Insufficient knowledge and experience in working with multiproblem individuals can, in turn, influence staff attitudes and willingness to reach out to resistant and/or ambivalent clients. The dilemma is that the mental health professional may tend, as Scherl points out, "to respond to his lack of understanding of the patient, and the overwhelming nature of the problems faced by the patient, with feelings of helplessness leading to anger and guilt. Both patient and professional can become trapped in their mutual sense of inadequacy to cope with these problems, and as a result, communication never gets established, or breaks down quickly if it does." [5] In this regard, Homonoff comments that: "The mistrust, hopelessness, and alienation felt by many white middle-class workers when faced by poor clients (especially black or Spanish-speaking) can cause them to give up with these clients and eventually 'cool them out' of the agency." [1] The thrust of service delivery is narrowed to those clients who are motivated enough to continue seeking out treatment on their own. As a result, as Macht suggests, "to the poor and minority groups, they [CMHCs] frequently appear alien, distant, establishmentarian, and not relevant." [2] Given the training deficits and the service commitments of community mental health center staff, outreach and advocacy services have received low priority.

By virtue of community participation in the development of policy and of geographic proximity, neighborhood health centers have special opportunities to provide outreach and advocacy services on a continuing basis. One major problem preventing this development has been the availability and use of mental health services to date. According to Macht, "Until recently mental health services in neighborhood health centers have been nonexistent or poorly integrated into the overall functioning of the centers."[2] Problems of internal fragmentation of services frequently extend to other disciplines as well, hindering the development of staff allegiances to a coordinated, interdisciplinary approach to service delivery.

For most neighborhood health centers, however, the overriding issue most affecting the extent and flexibility of service delivery has been financial. Faced with dwindling federal and state funding, the staff of neighborhood health centers have had to intensify their efforts to produce clinical encounters in the center in order to increase third-party income. This, in turn, has diminished staff freedom to engage in such vital but basically nonreimbursable activities as case advocacy and interagency coordination of services. Insufficient income for staff salaries has also increased the dependence of neighborhood health centers on backup hospitals for part-time staff. Specifically in the area of mental health, the combination of institutional and health center responsibilities places serious limits on staff's flexibility and autonomy to develop a primary identity with the neighborhood and a thorough knowledge of its human services network. For mental health staff, many of whom have a limited framework of training and experience working in low-income neighborhoods, time restrictions and the emphasis on producing health-center based clinical encounters often results in a narrow focus and range of service delivery. Without the opportunity and the encouragement to broaden their neighborhood perspective and establish collaborative linkage with other neighborhood providers, mental health staff run the risk of providing traditional community mental health services in a neighborhood health center setting. In the absence of coordinated strategies of neighborhood service intervention by health center staff, outreach and advocacy services are provided on a limited and individual case basis, primarily by noncredentialed staff members.

Some Advantages of the Outreach Model: Summary

One of the most significant features of the outreach model as developed by the JPOP is the emphasis on staff identification with, and commitment to, the Jamaica Plain neighborhood as a total system. Affiliated with backup institutions located outside the neighborhood, program staff were given the wide-ranging professional autonomy necessary to evolve their roles and provide services in response to neighborhood priorities. While the extent of staff independence was made possible in large part by the funding support of a federal staffing grant, an essential factor was the willingness of both backup institutions to support the concept of a grass roots mental health outreach program without imposing any preconceived institutional service priorities. Such a position served to heighten staff morale and allowed professional energy to focus on serving the neighborhood. Rather than perceiving themselves merely as extensions of the institutions, JPOP staff were able to view the institutions as one of several critical levels of service delivery available to better serve the neighborhood. Furthermore, this orientation allowed the JPOP staff to look primarily to the network of neighborhood human services providers rather than the institutions for emotional support, reward, and resources. As a result, the collaborative rather than dependent relationship that evolved between the JPOP and the backup institutions reduced significantly suspicions and expectations on all sides regarding such issues as staff support and program priority. Within the neighborhood itself, the JPOP's gradual establishment of multiple, grass roots service sites and affiliations emphasized the program's concern in playing a network-spanning role. Over a period of time, the free-floating orientation of the outreach team significantly enhanced both the staff's feelings and the perception of providers and consumers that the JPOP was an integral part of the neighborhood fabric.

The value of the outreach model lies in its ability to affect the delivery of services on different neighborhood levels and to avoid the liabilities usually associated with institution "satellite" programs, which are always considered low priority and second rate. Central to the model's approach is the broad base of linkages, with providers throughout the neighborhood. Collaboration with a range of neighborhood providers on an ongoing and informal basis provides the opportunity to develop systematic and coordinated approaches to early case finding, preventive intervention, and client care. Through the fostering of joint intervention strategies with other providers, the outreach team approach is able to seek out and engage many high-risk consumers outside the existing health care network.

With regard to client care, the emphasis of the outreach model is on extending support focused on the level of the client's expressed need. The informality, availability, and responsiveness of the outreach staff strongly counteract the fear and stigma many clients attach to mental health services provided in institutions. Therefore, when outreach counseling, case advocacy, and/or resource liaison services are offered, the site of service delivery is in the client's home or in an accommodating neighborhood base.

Finally, a vital impact of the outreach team approach is in the area of facilitating linkages among the various levels of the human services network. Building on a base of affiliations with backup institutions as well as collaborative neighborhood ties, the outreach model provides a framework for helping to establish comprehensive and integrated approaches of mental health care between a neighborhood and its surrounding community.

References

1. Homonoff, E., Community Casework and Clients' Rights. Unpublished manuscript, 1975.
2. Macht, L. B. Beyond the Mental Health Center: Planning for a Community of Neighborhoods. *Psychiatric Annals* 5:7 (July, 1975), 56-69.
3. Norman, M. M., Homonoff, E., and Hanson, G. Response to a Legislative Mandate: A Mental Health Model for Comprehensive School-Based Services to Inner-City Children with Special Needs. Paper presented at 52nd Annual Meeting, American Orthopsychiatric Association, Washington, D. C., 1975.
4. Scherl, D. J., and English, J. T. Community Mental Health and Comprehensive Health Service Programs for the Poor. *American Journal of Psychiatry.* 125:12 (June, 1969), 80-88.
5. Scherl, D. J. The Community Mental Health Center and Mental Health Services for the Poor. In H. Grunebaum (Ed.) *The Practice of Community Mental Health.* Little, Brown and Company, 1970, 171-195.

10

Linkages between Neighborhood Centers and Central Facilities

Orlando B. Lightfoot

As mental health programs decentralize to neighborhoods, the issue of linkage must be addressed and a view of services as linked parts of a system must be developed. The experience of the Boston University School of Medicine Division of Psychiatry in developing effective working alliances between its central facility and independent neighborhood centers is presented in this chapter as an illustration of planning and program operation in the area of linkages between neighborhood centers and central mental health facilities. Perhaps this work can shed light on the complexities of developing and sustaining these linkages which will be relevant to the other programs as well. Central facilities and neighborhood centers must be viewed as an integral part of a larger mental health network. Each subsystem within the total system is intimately linked and articulated with other subsystems. Alterations in administrative structure, budgetary allocation, program design, or philosophical orientation will greatly influence the quality and effectiveness of services delivered. This account, though documentary in nature, will not adhere strictly to historical sequence but will highlight and accentuate the development of adult ambulatory services. The term "ambulatory services" is used in a restricted manner to reflect outpatient psychiatric services, *excluding* programs for partial hospitalization, other alternatives to hospitalization, and programs for drug and alcohol abuse.

The geographic area to which the Solomon Carter Fuller Community Mental Health and Retardation Center (SCFMHC, formerly the Boston University Mental Health Center), Boston, Massachusetts, is responsible includes portions of four neighborhoods — Back Bay, the South End, Roxbury, and North Dorchester. This area of 115,000 people is ethnically diverse and includes blacks, whites, native Americans, Puerto Ricans, Orientals, and other ethnic groups. The region was designated a poverty area persuant to the 1970 amendment to the Community Mental Health and Retardation Center Construction and Staffing Act. [1]

Phase I — Neighborhood Centers and Psychiatric Practitioners

Four separate neighborhood centers began rudimentary programs in psychiatry before they were clearly aware of the status of the Solomon C. Fuller Mental Health and Retardation Center programs. Developing along different routes but each under the pressure of local community needs, the centers began in different parts of the catchment area (see Figures 10-1 and 10-2).

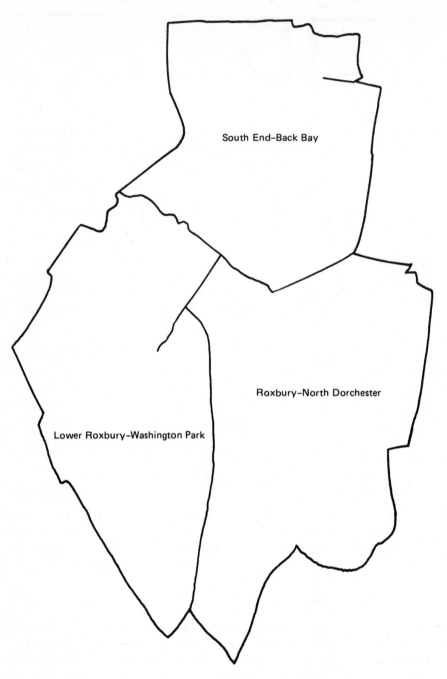

Figure 10-1. Schematic Diagram of Solomon C. Fuller Mental Health and Retardation Center Catchment Area (Boston, Massachusetts).

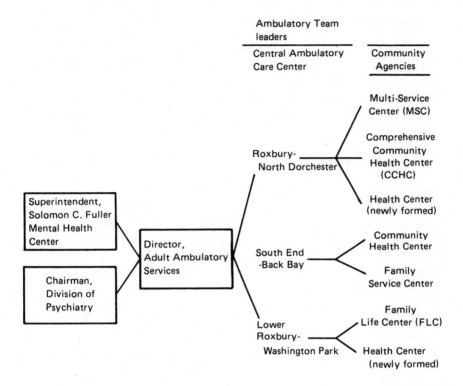

Figure 10-2. Organizational Chart Solomon C. Fuller Mental Health and
Retardation Center Ambulatory Program.

In Roxbury, to the east (in this chapter such designations of direction, refer
to parts of the Boston University Mental Health catchment area), a multiservice
center (MSC) was organized with specific focus on housing, social service, and
legal problems. Additionally, this center recognized the need for direct psychiatric patient/client care, as well as supervision and ongoing psychiatric consultation to the members of its primarily social service staff. A valued member of
the Division of Psychiatry faculty, a psychiatrist-psychoanalyst willing to utilize
his skills on somewhat less familiar turf, became the practitioner functioning in
this setting in 1965. He was willing to listen, learn, and modify his thinking and
interventions so that he could be useful to both the staff and the clients using
the multiservice center, who brought with them numerous housing, legal, and
complex social service problems. Over the next several years, he became an
important functioning cog in the intricate machinery that mobilized office and
home psychiatric care.

After a period of demonstrating his willingness to utilize his skills flexibly, his credibility was established, and he became the forerunner for future community and neighborhood mental health practitioners (staff and students) from the Division of Psychiatry. Each new person was thoroughly screened and accepted or rejected on the basis of their sensitivity to community needs, flexibility in applying their skills and willingness to work under the leadership of the multiservice center staff. This nuclear group became a loosely knit mental health team spending varying amounts of time at the multiservice center and the balance back at the specific units to which they were assigned within the Division of Psychiatry. They were a team only when assembled at the multiservice center and usually did not work there on the same day at the same time.

In Roxbury, also to the east, a comprehensive community health center (the RCCHC described in Chapter 8) began planning its mental health unit in 1968. This center, an OEO-funded facility, under the leadership of a project director, sought out and appointed a full-time psychiatrist. He was appointed to two departments simultaneously at the Boston University School of Medicine — the Department of Community Medicine and the Division of Psychiatry — and actively began to develop and implement a comprehensive program for the 38,000 residents within the comprehensive community health center's boundaries. As a full-time psychiatrist, he could develop a more intensive involvement and identification with the staff and various health team members, including social workers, community workers, nurses, and physicians. He became a health team member and provided continuity and follow-up on individual patients and their families. The program he conceived has since that time increased its initial staffing to include additional psychiatrists, psychologists, social workers, community workers, and nurses.

Roxbury's western region in the area called Lower Roxbury-Washington Park, lacked both a comprehensive multiservice center and a general health facility until planning began in 1968 for a Model Cities Family Life Center (FLC). The Chairman of the Division of Psychiatry, pleased by the success of the psychiatrist-psychoanalyst at the multiservice center, asked him to begin discussions with the appropriate Model Cities administration and consultants to organize a mental health unit. Having been sensitized somewhat to the complex issues involved, the psychiatrist helped develop a plan wherein a mental health team, originating out of the central facility at the mental health center, would be placed within the Family Life Center (FLC). This plan was greatly facilitated by the director of the Consultation and Education Program from which the mental health unit would be drawn. It was implemented with the placement of a consultation and education team consisting of a half-time psychiatrist, half-time social worker, and two community workers at the newly organized Family Life Center. The first year of the placement of the consultation and education team was a difficult one because, although there was agreement on the need for psychiatric input into the FLC, there was considerable disagreement as to the nature of the services to be provided. The consultation and education team's mandate was to provide consultation to the FLC staff as well as other agencies in the area. It was also to act as a conduit for referrals to the central facility at the mental health center. The staff at the FLC wanted all of this but felt direct patient evaluation and short-term treatment in the office or in the home was their greatest need. This difference in orientation concerning the function of the consultation and education team resulted in a withdrawal of the team from the FLC, producing a vacuum that was not readily filled.

The fourth neighborhood center to develop a mental health unit was a community health center in the South End. In 1970, the center hired a consultant-practitioner for one half-day per week. At the time the consultant-practitioner was hired, he was not a member of the Division of Psychiatry faculty, but later he was appointed to the faculty. His mandate at the health center was to assess the demand for mental health services of those patients already coming to the center in pediatrics and obstetrics and gynecology. He defined his role as a consultant to the staff and the administration, supervisor for those already dealing with the mental health needs of their patients, and direct service provider to children and their families in the office or in the home. This initial mandate was sanctioned by the community governing board of the center whose members insisted only that he maintain a high level of care, meet the patient in the setting most compatible with the patient's needs, and communicate to them at intervals on the development of the program. This service has developed to the point of currently having six part-time psychiatrists, two full-time psychologists, and one social worker, as well as a mental health administrative coordinator comprising the formal psychiatric cadre. The nurses and community health workers are an important part of this mental health effort.

Phase II - The Central Ambulatory Care Center and Linkages with Neighborhood Centers

The outpatient department of the Division of Psychiatry has evolved over the past 25 years from a small psychosomatic unit, to a more functional psychiatry clinic in 1959, to its present expanded form as an adult ambulatory service. The current administrative and functional arrangements reflect the expanded mandate of the unit, which now includes responsibility for patients referred from: (1) the University Hospital, (2) the catchment area, (3) the Boston University main campus, and (4) the Boston University Medical Center staff. The responsibility for a geographic area has strongly suggested the need for a more flexibly organized central facility which can readily respond to specific service requests and can be easily identified with a particular region of the service area (see Figures 10-1 and 10-2).

The central ambulatory care center has three functional ambulatory teams, each named and identified with a particular region of the service area. They are: the South End-Back Bay team, the Lower Roxbury-Washington Park team, and the Roxbury-North Dorchester team. These were originally formed by dividing the staff of the psychiatry clinic into thirds. The manpower pool which was divided included psychologists, social workers, nurses, community workers, and trainees in psychiatry, social work, and psychology. The number of staff in each discipline was not equal and, therefore, each team was not staffed in the same manner.

The first concrete linkage with a neighborhood center was made when the director of the mental health unit at the comprehensive community health center (CCHC) detailed above was appointed team leader of the Roxbury-North Dorchester team. Based primarily in a community center, it was anticipated that he could influence the development of the central unit in a particularly helpful manner, bringing with him the expertise gained in that center. He was also given the responsibility for consolidating all of the mental health activities occurring in the Roxbury-North Dorchester area, which included the unit at the multiservice center and a proposed unit at a newly developed health center. This linkage had the potential for integrating the staff of two separate organizations with different mandates and orientations. The problems of authority, responsibility, funding, allegiance, service obligations, training needs, responsibility to governing boards, and other crucial issues were dealt with by the top administrators of both institutions; and though not entirely resolved, this alliance was sanctioned. The newly appointed team leader then began to spend approximately one day per week functioning in his new capacity as team leader both in the neighborhood center and the central ambulatory care center.

His role up to the present time has been a difficult one, and many issues have surfaced, such as his commitment to each program and complaints by both staffs that he is not available enough. He has been unable to facilitate the movement of large numbers of staff between the two institutions, although some individuals have been extremely receptive. At the neighborhood center he must also contend with discipline boundaries between psychiatry, social service, and nursing, over which he has no administrative control. The first year of this linkage has made him aware of these issues, although no easy resolution is possible. The concept though is a viable one – functioning within and without – and this is the most important outcome of this linkage. These issues are similar and as complex in relation to the mental health unit at the multiservice center and the newly developed health center in the Roxbury East section.

As outlined in Phase I, the Model Cities Family Life Center had expressed a specific desire for direct patient care, brief evaluation and treatment, as well as consultation to the staff. The consultation and education team that had withdrawn from the FLC became an advocate for the FLC and also pointed out the need for these services. The Lower Roxbury-Washington Park ambulatory team responded to these requests by placing two team members in the FLC on a part-time basis. One staff psychiatrist and one third-year psychiatric resident became the link between the central ambulatory center and the neighborhood center. In addition, a community worker was used to coordinate this linkage around issues of records and facilitation of patient transfer between the neighborhood center and the central facility. The psychiatric personnel assigned to the FLC were regarded, after the usual period of suspicion and mistrust, as integral and important contributors to the health care team. This linkage was maintained for two years in its current form. It was severely affected by the withdrawal of all funding for the Model Cities health programs and the closing of the FLC. Many of the permanent staff of the FLC were absorbed into another health center which was in its initial operational stages in the Lower Roxbury-Washington Park section. The mental health unit was redeployed within the central ambulatory care center, and a fresh series of negotiations began with the health center just beginning in the Lower Roxbury-Washington Park area. The negotiations are not complete at this writing, but the hope remains that a mental health unit can be made operational within the near future.

The linkage in the South End-Back Bay region has been more difficult than anticipated. The team leader has been able to continue an ongoing alliance with the Family Service Center of a neighborhood social service agency. The Family Service Center has had a long-standing, direct service and supervisory relationship with a psychiatric consultant and those psychiatric residents working with him, but there has never been a formal relationship with the ambulatory services. A change in administrative leadership at the Family Service Center has delayed a more active alliance.

The team leader has not been able to effectively link the mental health unit at the Community Health Center in this area with the central ambulatory care center. The health center raises a number of objections to the placement of a team there. Staff feel that a situation in which individuals work in the health center but are paid by another source is not a desirable arrangement because of the issues of authority, responsibility, and allegiance. The center currently exercises, through its governing board, the final decision making power over hiring and firing and would not have that option if the person were paid by another organization. Health center staff are all concerned about the quality of care delivered by psychiatric residents — not that they are not capable, but if a placement is to be developed, they desire first a board-certified psychiatrist. They also express the view that some disciplines, particularly psychiatry, would be more helpful to their center than others, such as social service. The health center is beginning to soften on some of these issues as its association with residents and trainees in other health disciplines increases. Staff appropriately still insist on the delivery of service as the first priority, and teaching and training as very distant seconds. Through continued consultation with the administrators and clinicians at the central ambulatory center, some of the barriers are diminishing. This health center, though, poses very difficult questions that require continued attention.

Discussion

This chapter has presented one model for linking neighborhood and central facilities and raises several issues. The future of the programs discussed are in large measure dependent on the continued willingness of the administrative and clinical staffs within the neighborhood centers and the central ambulatory care center to continue the very active and oftimes difficult process involved in trying sensitively to provide quality care to all the patients in the service area. It requires careful and continuing evaluation and scrutiny of the individuals delivering service within these units. The very delicate mix between the delivery of service, teaching, and inservice training available for all staff—not simply trainees—must be continually titrated so that staff are stimulated to think, learn, and perform to their maximum capabilities.

The issue of authority and final decision-making power, so crucial to a truly community-controlled facility, must be handled in a manner that encourages well trained, sensitive staff to want to work and remain in neighborhood centers. This applies also to a central facility attempting to develop a community base.

In addition to attitudes, authority, and administrative difficulties, the issue of how services will be paid for is one that plagues and confounds the entire health system. It is becoming increasingly important that each person requiring service have some ability to defray expenses for that service. This makes the issue of third-party payment one that may cause linkages such as the ones begun in the previous account unworkable. If both the neighborhood center and the central ambulatory care center are actively competing for the same third-party dollar, one or the other unit will suffer. It will not be possible to simply look to the federal government for a solution. The answers are not certain, but the need for continued services remain. A number of possibilities are currently under consideration, including contracts between the central facility and the neighborhood centers. This arrangement would allow a pooling of resources and foster a fiscal cooperation that maximizes the advantages of either the central facility or the neighborhood center. Creative alliances between the central facility and the centers and other health providers, such as hospitals and nursing homes, may be the future direction.

The Division of Psychiatry is using the building blocks of the ambulatory teams as a nidus for more comprehensive clinical units that relate an inpatient ward, a consultation and education team, an emergency team, and a partial hospitalization team. These separate units, if linked under one administrative and clinical leader, could lead to more flexible use of the treatment options available for a patient in need during a crisis and for continuity afterward. It is apparent from the first year of planning for this modular structure that it depends on a commitment of resources for administration, a willingness to share and possibly shift power and authority alliances, and a philosophical orientation that will allow the idea to develop into a reality. As of this writing, the modular approach remains a useful idea, but full implementation is still in the distant future.

Conclusions

The experiences of the Division of Psychiatry have highlighted a number of important issues.

1. Linkages between systems are best formed and more easily maintained if each independent system is relatively stable. A clear distinction, though, must be made between a stable system and a static one (i.e., central ambulatory services and community centers, respectively).
2. Stability within a system, and thus between systems, is enhanced by adequate staffing, continuous funding, and creative leadership.
3. Linkages between systems can best be made if a facilitator is involved who is familiar with aspects of both systems. This person can often help minimize distortions, modulate projections, and foster creative alliances (for example, the psychiatrist-psychoanalyst from the Division of Psychiatry).
4. Certain conflicts are entirely expectable and consistently present when linking independent systems. Conflicts over opposing mandates and basic philosophical orientation; issues of authority, control and responsibility; pooling of resources and sharing dividends: all of these issues are fundamental when even considering a linkage between systems (such as the health center in the South End, the comprehensive community health center, and a modular structure).

Many issues are yet to be resolved and require continuous dialogue and monitoring for the future. Community-based neighborhood centers and centrally located ambulatory centers are both structures for the present and for the future. Their form and direction will evolve over time as a function of the dynamic past.

Our notion of linkage, shared by others with similar approaches [2,3,4], clearly implies a systems orientation to the delivery of mental health services wherein separate levels of service delivery, from inpatient through neighborhood based programs, are joined to serve a discrete geographic area.

References

1. United States Congress, Public Law 91-211, Amendment for an Act, United States Government Printing Office, 1970.

2. Cohen, R.E. "Development of the Interface Team in the Harbor Area Mental Health Program." Unpublished manuscript.

3. Macht, L.B., "Beyond the Mental Health Center: Planning for a Community of Neighborhoods," *Psychiatric Annals*, Vol. 5, No. 7, July, 1975.

4. _____, "On Community-Based Care," *Psychiatric Annals*, Vol. 4, No. 6, June, 1974.

Part III

Neighborhood Psychiatry: Research and Training

Introduction

Having defined a context in Part I and described specific program models and issues in Part II, this section turns to research and training issues in neighborhood psychiatry, and includes chapters which review conceptual questions as well as matters of operational detail. The first portion of Part III deals with research issues, the second with training; within each subportion, discussion proceeds from general matters to more specific ones.

We view research and training as critical to both the development and the evaluation of the field, and as basic to setting directions for the future. If a large pool of neighborhood-based workers is to be created, it will require both the education of students just starting out, and the reeducation and in-service training of established workers. As can be readily seen from the preceding two sections, new roles and functions have arisen and a cadre of new practitioners must be trained. These practitioners must be educated in applicable special techniques beyond the usual basic mental health skills. They should know, as well, how to function in a relevant, useful, and acceptable fashion in neighborhood settings. Further, if the field is to survive, a body of skills and knowledge must be distilled from the experience of the initial practitioners, documented, taught to the next generation of workers, and subjected to evaluation.

The section opens with a consideration by Klerman and Borus of the conceptual issues facing research in this field. They discuss the importance for the researcher of an understanding of the target neighborhood. They review some recent studies and propose strategies for collaboration between researchers and neighborhood residents and for research implementation. Along with Beck and Long in the chapter following, they point clearly to the importance of neighborhood sensitivities when research is contemplated and performed. Often local suspicion arises, with neighborhood residents concerned about being "ripped off" by researchers whose studies "do nothing for the neighborhood." Neighborhood-based research fares best if it evolves from a base of neighborhood service and an ongoing commitment to the neighborhood. Issues of service delivery, for example, can be examined to the neighborhood's benefit by documenting services, needs, costs, and outcome.

Beck and Long, in their chapter, provide a detailed design for the evaluation of neighborhood mental health services and a way of comparing those services, along a number of dimensions, with other ambulatory psychiatric services. The study they describe could be performed as a whole or in parts by others and provides the reader with a blueprint for such evaluative research which could be adapted readily to a variety of different settings. Work of this kind could produce comparative data crucial for program planning, development, evaluation, and accountability.

The results of an evaluative study of a neighborhood mental health service by Leopold and Kluft concludes the research and evaluation portion of this section. The study documents the importance of locally integrated and comprehensive service delivery as a key to effectiveness. The chapter illustrates how evaluative research can simultaneously be used for purposes of program assessment and program development. In so doing, Leopold and Kluft demonstrate in practice the conceptual notions of Klerman and Borus and elements of the design proposed by Beck and Long.

The section next considers a panoply of education and training issues. Fox begins with a description of mental health skill training for a variety of neighborhood workers based on principles of adult learning. From a description of a particular program, she extrapolates a series of basic principles for education in neighborhood psychiatry and for training the trainers of neighborhood practitioners. This is especially critical in a new field such as this in which, in addition to the overwhelming needs for training existing workers, a new cadre of teachers must also be developed. Sharfstein and Sabin then follow with a chapter briefly outlining issues of psychiatric residency training in neighborhood settings. The specific concerns they raise, however, are not unique to psychiatry. All neighborhood training must deal with questions of cost, the trade-off between service and teaching, the follow-up of trainees, and the identity issues which must be faced and resolved if future practitioners of neighborhood psychiatry are to emerge.

Part III concludes with a chapter by Jiminez which focuses specifically on a training program in neighborhood mental health for workers in Hispanic neighborhoods. This chapter offers not only a particular example of such a training program but also a generic format for locally sensitive training in neighborhood work. It presents ways for dealing with supervisor/supervisee conflict in these settings, group process, and didactic issues. In addition, it presents a particular schema for understanding the adjustment patterns of Spanish-speaking (and other) neighborhood immigrants. Jiminez suggests the use of an experiential training method which he developed and which he offers as one paradigm for training in neighborhood psychiatry.

11

Research and Evaluation in Neighborhood Mental Health

Gerald L. Klerman and
Jonathan F. Borus

Neighborhood mental health is a relatively new and evolving delivery system in the United States. It represents a progressive modification of the community mental health movement of the sixties, focusing the former's population orientation onto smaller and more realistically sized ethnic or destiny related, geographic areas [1]. As seen in the chapters describing program models, neighborhood mental health services are usually structured as an integral component of a comprehensive neighborhood health or human services system [2]. It is hoped that delivery of mental health services within such comprehensive, consumer-influenced neighborhood settings will provide a better quality of ambulatory care than the larger, free-standing community mental health center.

However, mental health services, together with other components of human services, are under increasing public scrutiny and criticism [3,4]. In this context, the proponents of new approaches, such as those embodied in neighborhood mental health systems, can expect searching questions to be asked by citizens, consumers, legislators, and other professionals. Anticipating the likely competition among various services for the increasingly scarce public dollar, research and evaluation have vital functions [5]. Knowledge is power, and the absence of evaluation data and knowledge can render programs and program administrators powerless. The advocates of neighborhood mental health services in the seventies would do well to look at the experiences of publicly funded human service programs of the sixties, such as manpower training, community action programs, and other service systems. High expectations were generated for amelioration of important social problems, followed by periods of disillusionment and criticism in which the program leaders were unable to provide adequate data to document the extent to which the hopes, expectations, and claims with which their programs were initiated had been realized in practice [6].

To date, evaluative research of neighborhood mental health has been quite limited and quantitative studies are still in the planning stage. Two recent reports from studies of 19 neighborhood-health-center-based mental health programs in Boston present an aggregate assessment of the qualitative advantages and problems of neighborhood mental health. The first of these reports [7] describes four different organizational models of neighborhood mental health programs determined by the differing contributions to these programs of the overlapping neighborhood health and community mental health systems. The strategic position of neighborhood mental health programs at the interface of these two systems was reported to have enabled them to develop a variety of internal linkages to primary health providers and external linkages to community mental health and other neighborhood caregivers. The internal linkages to primary health providers were seen as faciliating necessary communication about patient care for referral, consultation, and collaborative efforts; improving the success of referrals without "loss" of the patient between referring and referred caregivers; and promoting coordinated planning of physical and mental health care. External linkages allowed the neighborhood and community mental health programs to complement rather than compete with each other in order to provide a broad spectrum of mental health care. Mechanisms and problems in maintaining collaborative rather than competitive linkages between systems were described.

The second report [8] described the services provided by these neighborhood health center mental health programs and some of the effects of delivering ambulatory mental health services as part of a primary health care system. Staff utilization data from these programs showed that most of their efforts focused on the provision of direct mental health services to neighborhood residents and indirect consultative and collaborative services to general health staff to facilitate the coordination of health care. Data were presented to support hypotheses that mental health services provided in a primary health care setting are geographically and culturally accessible and psychologically acceptable. These programs served a disproportionately high percentage of children, and almost a quarter of all services were provided in outreach visits, primarily in patients' homes. Benefit within a conjoint primary health-mental health delivery site derived from early case finding, successful referral, and coordination of general health services; 48 percent of the referrals for mental health services in these programs were of patients first identified and referred by the general health staff at the conjoint health-mental health delivery site. There is evidence that these services compliment and add to the efficiency of a comprehensive primary health care delivery system. Both papers provide a review of persistent problem areas for neighborhood-health-center-based mental health programs and describe areas of needed quantitative evaluation of such delivery systems.

It is therefore both a challenge and a necessity for the fledgling field of neighborhood mental health to closely evaluate its precepts and programs as it develops. In this chapter we will focus on salient conceptual issues underlying delivery of mental health services at the neighborhood level, delineate research and evaluation questions which derive from these issues, describe a strategy for professional-consumer collaboration in these investigations, and comment on some expectable tactical problems in pursuing evaluation efforts which are consequences of the unique aspects of the neighborhood concept.

Some Salient Conceptual Issues

In discussing the salient issues for research and evaluation, we have chosen to focus on testing the theoretical bases for the unique aspects of neighborhood mental health. The emergence of these efforts in the past decade arose from the widely discussed crisis in urban life and the desire to restructure the delivery patterns of human services, including health, housing, public safety, and education, to provide for decentralized and locally oriented systems for the delivery of service [9].

The rationale for this approach was based on a number of accepted conclusions about social change and urban life in the latter third of the twentieth century. Migration to the cities, displacement from family homes by urban renewal, residential mobility, and the rapid disappearance of the extended family and other structures of social organization in communities have been shown to relate to an increased sense of social isolation, anomie and, perhaps, increased rates of mental illness [10,11,12,13]. Today, over three fourths of the population of the United States lives in urban settings. With the growth of urban settings and the attendant concentration of populations, a breakdown has occurred in the organization and cohesion of community life, as well as the informal, face-to-face networks of social participation and control. Toennies, the nineteenth-century German sociologist, contrasted *Gemeinschaft* communities, organized around face-to-face contact, common values, and informal modes of control, with *Gesellschaft* communities, organized on an impersonal level around formal vertical hierarchies [14]. The rapid changes in our society have decreased the number of *Gemeinschaft* communities, producing urban areas today which are organized primarily in a *Gesellschaft* manner.

Panzetta [15] has pointed out that the community mental health movement has been "short circuited" by confusion between these two concepts of community; although community mental health theory rests on a *Gemeinschaft* organization of communities, the application of this theory to the delivery of mental health services has often floundered when applied to the large, unintegrated *Gesellschaft* "catchmented communities" mandated by the federal funding legislation as the basic units of service delivery.

Neighborhood mental health is an attempt to further decentralize the delivery of mental health services by decreasing the size of the population served by the delivery system, focusing on a smaller, more interrelated *Gemeinschaft* level of organization, more actively involving the consumer of services in determining the priorities of service delivery, and providing a more comprehensive scope of health and other human services within the same delivery system.

The ultimate test of any mental health delivery system is to see if it works— that is, if its services decrease the manifestation of and disability from mental illness in the population served [16]. In determining whether neighborhood mental health works, two prominent hypotheses can be tested. First, can the neighborhood delivery system decrease mental illness by providing more effective direct and indirect mental health services. Second, can a neighborhood delivery system in itself help produce better organized *Gemeinschaft* communities by increasing citizen participation, cohesion, and leadership to provide a counterforce against the isolation, anomie, impersonality, and the social disorganization associated with increased mental illness. Yates, in a paper entitled "Neighborhood Government," identified four possible results of the decentralization of numerous urban human services which lend support to this second hypothesis [17]. To paraphrase Yates, decentralization will:

1. increase the responsiveness of administrative units and agencies to local neighborhood needs;
2. reduce the felt and perceived "distance" between citizens, agencies, and government, and, consequently, increase citizens' feelings of efficacy as participants in the political and social process;
3. facilitate increased community cohesion, thereby, focusing local resources and concern on shared priorities and problems; and
4. increase the resources of local democracy by contributing to the development of local leaders and by providing for wider opportunities for citizen involvement in decision making.

Decentralization of services to the neighborhood level will in this view increase citizen participation, cohesion, and leadership, influencing not only the political process but also the social organization within the neighborhood, and thus also positively influencing the mental health behaviors and potentials of neighborhood residents.

Research Questions

To examine these two hypotheses, research is needed into the delivery of services, the coordination of services, the impact of the delivery system on the neighborhood, and the costs of services. Each of these areas raises a number of research questions, and we do not imply that these are the only research questions or even the most researchable ones. However, they give some indication of the areas of inquiry in which development of meaningful outcome measures is necessary. (The reader is also referred to the chapter by Beck and Long for a further discussion of some of these issues.)

Delivery of Services

A primary research task is to determine if districting at the neighborhood level improves the accessibility, acceptability, and fruitful utilization of services by consumers. Questions include: What services are most appropriately delivered at the neighborhood level? Who will be reached by such a delivery system and who will be excluded? Are there neighborhood-specific crises which precipitate illness? How does delivery of mental health services at the neighborhood level compare in terms of accessability, acceptability, and utilization with alternative delivery systems, such as private practice and free-standing community mental health centers? Does a neighborhood or districted model of service delivery work in organized as well as disorganized, rich as well as poor, private-practitioner-served as well as private-practitioner-deprived neighborhoods?

Coordination of Services

A second research area must ascertain if the neighborhood system increases the coordination of caregiving agencies in the neighborhood to avoid caregiver conflict and duplication of, or gaps in, service. How does integration with a comprehensive health care system increase quality integration and continuity of total health care? Will mental health care delivered at the neighborhood level increase the availability and coordination of other public and private caregivers—private sectors of medicine and psychiatry, welfare agencies, family service agencies, and public health agencies—to those citizens with emotional difficulties as components of multiproblem situations? Will a mental health care delivery system which is an integral part of a general health or social service network reach people in need earlier in their illness? Since neighborhood mental health currently coexists with larger, governmentally sanctioned and funded community mental health systems, what will be the effects on utilization patterns and on preferences for services, or on integration or duplication of services when there are multiple portals of entry into the delivery system? What will be effective patterns of administrative liaison and coordination of the neighborhood and community delivery systems to provide continuity of care and a full range of ambulatory and hospital mental health services?

Impact on the Neighborhood

A third research area focuses on understanding the impact and effect of the service delivery system on the neighborhood itself. Can neighborhood delivery of health and mental health services increase neighborhood organization and cohesion as has been suggested? If so, what are meaningful measures of neighborhood organization? Does such a delivery system increase community acceptance and readiness to actively deal with the chronically ill in the neighborhood setting? To avoid the therapeutically empty transfer of such patients from the back wards of our hospitals to the back alleys of our neighborhoods, can neighborhood mental health provide integrated local support systems for the productive, community-based maintenance of the psychiatrically disabled? Will these new service delivery systems help define a more functional consumer constituency in the neighborhood to work cooperatively with professionals?

Costs

Regarding finances: Can such a system be cost-effective, self supporting, and prevent costly hospitalization? How do the costs and benefits compare with other systems of care? How do we analyze all of the costs of neighborhood services as well as analyze the complex benefits embodied in our hypotheses stated earlier?

These specific research areas and questions in the field of neighborhood mental health provide broad programmatic scope for possible research. Attention is now directed to some unique issues in approaching the neighborhood for purposes of developing a research alliance.

A Strategy for Professional-Consumer Collaboration

In many neighborhoods served by neighborhood health and mental health centers, research and evaluation are words and concepts charged with negative affect. The common values, mutual dependence, and horizontal relationships characteristic of the *Gemeinschaft* aspect of many of these neighborhoods have been maintained by forced isolation and, at times, oppression of the usually poor, minority group inhabitants [15]. "Research" connotes exploitation by outsiders (often the professional investigators themselves) and use as guinea pigs for others' benefit. "Evaluation" is a slightly more acceptable concept, if it is seen as important to understanding and improving the provision of services to the neighborhood.

Most neighborhood health or multiservice centers, as joint efforts of non-neighborhood professionals and neighborhood consumers, implicitly encourage the face-to-face relationships and active consumer participation characteristic of *Gemeinschaft* organization. Although the mental health professionals are most often self- or consumer-designated to conduct the "formal" research and evaluation of a center's mental health program, if meaningful data are to be obtained in such efforts, mental health professionals must gain the sanction of the consumers and work out a strategy for collaboration with consumer representatives in the research and evaluation planning, process, and feedback.

Gaining the sanction of neighborhood consumers for operational research and evaluation should be facilitated by the smaller size and *Gemeinschaft* nature of the neighborhood delivery system. Defining consumer representatives who speak with and to some extent can speak for the neighborhood is always a difficult task, but is made easier if shared values and horizontal communication networks function in the neighborhood. Consumer representatives, usually coalesced as a neighborhood health center board of directors or consumer board, are often stimulated to participate in planning studies which will feed back to them a better understanding of the care presently provided and delineate areas for improvement of the services provided in their neighborhood. They also are keenly aware that such studies are helpful and often essential in justifying funding requests to provide care for the consumers they represent.

In our experience, consumer representatives at the neighborhood level of service delivery have a genuine and immediate interest in the quality of care provided by the center to themselves, their relatives, and good friends. At the interface between the care providers and the care consumers, these representatives on the neighborhood board receive informal evaluation of the neighborhood mental health services from both the direct and indirect consumers of this care. This informal feedback of consumers' appraisals of service from their individual perceptions and experiences with the delivery system may raise issues in need of more comprehensive investigation in a formal manner. Because of this interface position, the input of the consumer representatives into the planning process of research and evaluation should help define areas and methods of investigation which will be meaningful and acceptable to the neighborhood.

In presenting an initial investigation proposal to a consumer board, the professionals should adopt a straightforward "something for something" approach, emphasizing both costs and beneifts of the project to the consumers of service, the neighborhood board, and the professionals. The day has long since passed when consumers will naively accept research as an unexplained adjunct to receiving medical and mental health care. An explanation of the short- and long-range reasons for the investigation are essential and productive in working out a collaborative project with a consumer board. The consumer board can then evaluate the proposal and suggest tactical modifications to improve its neighborhood relevance and acceptability. The "something for something" approach recognizes the realistic interdependence of the providers and consumers of care, and the insufficiency of either alone to evaluate the success or failure of a program.

Tactical Problems

In pursuing the above strategy for research and evaluation of neighborhood mental health services, we have become aware of tactical problems which are themselves consequences of *Gemeinschaft* aspects of the neighborhood concept. Tactically, evaluative efforts should not impede service provision, frighten or coerce consumers, threaten paraprofessional service providers, or ignore neighborhood values and consumer board responsibilities.

The investigation should be designed so that it does not inhibit the accessibility of neighborhood mental health care services to the consumer. The provision of mental health care services within a neighborhood health center allows patients the unique opportunity to "slide over" from the general health to mental health area of responsibility without defining themselves as mentally ill or as mental health patients. Toward the same end, neighborhood mental health workers often make the initial contact with the patient in nontraditional settings, such as the home, in other community agencies, or in the general health component of the neighborhood health center. This avoidance of self-labeling or neighborhood stigma is one of the attractive advantages to many citizens seeking mental health care in a comprehensive health setting, and for many it increases their accessibility to and acceptability of services. To avoid the creation of barriers to service, research forms or questionnaires should not confront patients with inquiries which force definition of their problems as emotional, and may thus identify and potentially stigmatize the patient as "mentally ill" in the eyes of his neighbors. In poorer neighborhoods, written questionnaires requesting demographic data may also be seen as a threat to confidentiality and/or needed welfare benefits, thereby inhibiting accessibility to service and the building of a therapeutic alliance.

Research and evaluation efforts should not frighten or coerce consumers of care into passive-aggressive responses. Many of the consumers of neighborhood mental health services have previously utilized the public sector of the health care system and often in the past have felt covertly coerced to participate in research efforts as a payment for service. There is strong concern that the neighborhood health center patient not be coerced by professionals or by habit to pay for his service through participation in research that will not benefit him either directly, by influencing *his* care, or indirectly, by influencing the quality of care in the center as a whole. Especially in as subjective an area as mental health, patients who feel coerced will often comply in a passive aggressive or hostile manner, resulting in the evaluation effort generating data of questionable value.

Evaluation is also threatening to the indigenous paraprofessional caregivers who operate under considerable role strain in providing much of the neighborhood mental health care. Midway between the consumer and the professional, with little institutional history to their role identity, they fear being caught between the often differing expectations of the consumers and professionals and being held responsible for gaps in the program. They also fear that research and evaluation efforts may intrude on their informal, "citizen to citizen" approach with patients by formalizing their role and detrimentally increasing the distance between them and their patients.

Lastly, it is important to carefully define with the consumer board the type of evaluation feedback which will be most meaningful and useful to their constituents. Both the consumer board member's role as program priority setter and the confidentiality of information about fellow-citizen patients must be respected in this process.

The negative aspects of these considerations need not ultimately preclude research development. Rather, an understanding of their existence, operation, and intimate relationship to the cohesive nature of a *Gemeinschaft* community which neighborhood mental health attempts to facilitate should help to foster rational planning of research to ensure its acceptance, relevance, and success.

Conclusions

For neighborhood mental health, research and evaluation cannot be a luxury to be appended to the end of a budget request in order to assuage state or federal funding guidelines. Rather, a systematic program for the generation of information to increase theoretical understanding in this new field and to assess the relative efficacy and cost efficiency of its programs is necessary for its survival and long-term growth and expansion. If proponents of new neighborhood mental health programs ignore the failure of earlier efforts to document theoretical and programmatic claims, they too may be destined to reap similar difficulties and despair.

References

1. Macht, L.B. "Neighborhood Psychiatry." *Psychiatric Annals, 4:9*, September, 1974.
2. Morrill, R.G. "A New Mental Health Services Model for the Comprehensive Neighborhood Health Center." *American Journal of Public Health, 62*: 1108-1111, 1972.
3. Klerman, G.L. "Public Trust and Professional Confidence." *Smith College Studies in Social Work*, February: 115-124, 1972.
4. Arnhoff, F.N. "Social Consequences of Policy Toward Mental Illness." *Science, 188*: 1277-1281, 1975.
5. Klerman, G.L. "Current Evaluation Research on Mental Health Services." *American Journal of Psychiatry, 131*: 783-787, 1974.
6. Moynihan, D. *Maximum Feasible Misunderstanding: Community Action in the War on Poverty.* New York: The Free Press, 1969.
7. Borus, J.F., Janowitch, L.A., Kieffer, F., Morrill, R.G., Reich, L, Simone, E., Towle, L. "The Coordination of Mental Health Services at the Neighborhood Level." *American Journal of Psychiatry, 132*: 1177-1181, 1975.
8. Borus, J.F. "Neighborhood Health Centers as Providers of Primary Mental Health Care." *New England Journal of Medicine*, in press 1976.
9. Klerman, G.L. "Mental Health and the Urban Crisis." *American Journal of Orthopsychiatry, 39*: 818-826, October, 1969.

10. Lindemann, E. "Mental Health and the Environment." In: *The Urban Condition*, Duhl, L.J. (ed.). New York: Basic Books, Inc. 3-10, 1963.

11. Fried, M. "Grieving for a Lost Home." In: *The Urban Condition*, Duhl, Leonard J. (ed). New York: Basic Books, Inc., 151-171, 1963.

12. Strole, L., Michael, S.T., Langer, T.S., Opler, M.D., and Rennie, T.A.C. *Mental Health in the Metropolis: The Midtown Manhattan Study*. New York: Blackiston, 1962.

13. Leighton, A.H. *My Name is Legion*. New York: Basic Books, Inc. 1959.

14. Nisbet, R.A. *The Sociological Tradition*. New York: Basic Books, Inc. 1966.

15. Panzetta, A.F. "The Concept of Community: The Short-Circuit of the Mental Health Movement." *Archives of General Psychiatry*, *25*: 291-297, 1971.

16. Wing, J.D. "Principles of Evaluation." In: *Evaluating a Community Psychiatric Service*, Wing, J.K., Hailey, Anthea M. (eds.). London: Oxford Univ. Press, 11-39, 1972.

17. Yates, D. "Neighborhood Government." *Policy Sciences, 3*: 209-217, 1972.

12

Evaluation of Mental Health Services in a Neighborhood Health Center

James C. Beck and
Jancis V.F. Long

Over the past fifteen years, recognition of the importance of evaluation research as a tool for assessing mental health service programs has increased. Many articles and books [1-9] have been written elaborating conceptual schemes for evaluation research, addressing methodological issues, discussing practical political implications, and repeatedly stressing the value of doing such research. The theoretical issues of evaluation have been addressed in the mental health literature so frequently that the author of a recent article [10] suggested that evaluators of other medical care services should consult the mental health evaluation literature for approaches to the conceptualization and resolution of evaluation problems in medical care delivery. Other articles report on the results of program evaluations actually carried out, ranging from short summaries of the results of implementing particular changes in some form of service delivery [11-13] to massive reports on entire systems [14]. What is not immediately apparent from the literature is how the administrator or chief of evaluation in a given system should proceed if he or she wants to design a study to learn about the effectiveness and efficiency of the service being provided as compared to alternative types of service delivery.

This chapter presents an actual protocol for what we believe to be a feasible and useful research project. It may also be read as a check list of variables to be considered, or as a set of methodological suggestions for people designing their own evaluation research. For this purpose, reference is made to key articles in the literature in which issues raised are discussed in greater detail. Though the suggested project in its entirety would clearly require significant funding, we have indicated various ways in which the scope could be reduced to focus on specific questions. Such partial studies could be carried out with relatively small budgets.

Mental Health in Neighborhood Health Centers

Since the first OEO-funded neighborhood health centers began to operate in 1966, mental health professionals have seen a new opportunity to deliver mental health services. It is the clear impression of professionals working in such facilities that they offer services to people who would not be served by other programs, even those such as community mental health centers, in which cost is not a barrier. In particular, the lives of many people with little money or education, with poor jobs or no jobs, are seen as bound to a large extent to their neighborhoods. It is said that these people will not travel out of their neighborhood for health care except under extreme duress and will be quite unwilling to seek psychiatric assistance outside the neighborhood. When such people develop serious mental illnesses or decompensate during normal life crises, they are not liable to seek professional attention unless it is available close to home. The importance of distance relative to other factors in determining utilization of health care facilities has been contested, but it is clearly important. Collver [15], for example, claimed distance was of primary importance in determining use of services, while so many authors have challenged this that McKinlay [16] has noted: "Despite widespread knowledge that geographical considerations are not the only or necessarily the most important determinants of utilization, the concept of the neighborhood health center is espoused in the United States and in Great Britain as a means of meeting the emerging health needs of certain populations." However, in addition to the issue of distance from clients, evidence suggests that the community-based, relatively small-sized neighborhood health center is conducive to developing new, more constructive staff attitudes toward and understanding of patients. And this may well be as important in encouraging utilization as geographic proximity [17].

Evaluation of What for Whom?

Anyone designing a research project for evaluation of service should be very clear about who wants the research done and for what kinds of decisions the information is to be used. Some administrators, for example, mainly want a good description of the way a service functions, with aggregate figures about who uses it, for how long, patient contacts per staff member, staff contacts per patient, and so forth. From this kind of data the administrator can form his or her own conclusions about the kind of evaluative research most appropriate for the service, and may require from the original descriptive study no more than a paragraph of ideas about the directions further study could take. Other administrators want to know how good a given service is, considered along various dimensions; they want evidence of problematic or successful service on which to base future decisions about funding, staffing, and training.

For a complete evaluation of a service three basic steps are necessary:

1. An answer to the question, "What's going on here?", in terms of a thorough description as indicated above.

2. An answer to the question, "What should be going on here?", in terms of criteria for quality of service along various dimensions.

3. An answer to the question, "How good is what is going on here?", in terms of an analysis of how well a service meets specified criteria.

A fourth step which is not logically necessary but may in fact be the most useful is:

4. An attempt to answer the question, "What can be done about improving what is going on here?"

The research schema described in this chapter would produce a reasonably complete answer to (1) and partial answers to (2) and (3). A thorough description of a neighborhood health center would be complete, while the similar descriptions of other ambulatory mental health services would yield the comparative material from which reasonable criteria could be *generated*. The data would be sufficiently detailed to be used to complete (3) and (4) when the criteria were decided on. This schema does not provide the criteria.

Another area not covered by this material is that of cost efficiency. For this important aspect we refer evaluators to some publications where the issues and techniques of cost accounting in medical care are presented [18-22]. Much of the data to be gathered in the proposed study could be used as measures of benefit in a cost-benefit analysis of a neighborhood health center. We suggest also that anyone attempting a cost-benefit study consult with a local private health maintenance organization or prepaid group practice that provides mental health care. Cost accounting in these organizations is very highly developed because it is essential to their continued operation.

We would like to stress, therefore, that though we frequently use the term "evaluation research," this study would *give the administrator the detailed descriptive material on which an evaluation could be based*; it would also serve to locate specific problems and provide background for policy-making to solve them.

Outline of a Study

The following study suggests that a body of comparable detailed information about delivery of mental health services be gathered for a neighborhood health center and four other types of facilities serving similar or comparable populations. The other facilities are: (1) general hospital emergency rooms; (2) psychiatry outpatient clinics in general hospitals; (3) free-standing ambulatory mental health facilities; (4) health maintenance organizations. Although health maintenance organizations differ from the other facilities in that they are invariably private and typically do not provide health services to people who cannot afford to pay the full cost, they are included for comparison because there is a good possibility that they will become the model for delivery of all kinds of ambulatory health services in the future.

We suggest three different simultaneous methods for gathering data from the five facilities. (These are described briefly here and more detailed protocols are provided in the final section of this chapter in Appendix 12A.) These are:

1. A descriptive study of services offered, utilization of services, and characteristics of utilizers at each of the five types of facility.

2. An intensive sample survey in which patient/staff sessions are observed by independent research interviewers, and follow-up interviews are conducted with both staff and patients. By interviewing patients at the beginning of a service episode and again later, one can assess the benefit or lack of it associated with their contact with the facility. Moreover, in this way patients' views of the quality of service they received can be obtained. Only by observing staff at their work can an assessment of the quality of their clinincal work and an understanding of what they are trying to do with patients be made.

3. A staff interaction study in which a researcher spends all of several working days with each of several staff members at all the facilities. In this way a researcher can assess the actual level of collaboration and consultation that takes place with staff members of the facilities, and between one facility staff and others. We think that self-reports, or questionnaires regarding either direct service or indirect service, are not adequate substitutes for careful observation by an independent researcher.

Although the comparative nature of this research would give valuable depth and perspective to the information provided from any one facility, the study could be reduced in scope by reducing the number of facilities to be compared. Even limiting it to a single neighborhood health center (NHC) would produce a thorough description, though with little potential for generating criteria or suggesting directions for improvement. The project could be further reduced in scope by attempting only one or two of the three proposed methods of gathering data.

This study is largely intended to provide descriptive parametric data for use in developing criteria and evaluating the comparative effectiveness of a given sample of mental health care programs. However, the testing of specific hypotheses could easily be incorporated within it. For instance, the claim that neighborhood health centers attract many people who would not otherwise become consumers of mental health services would be tested by checking whether neighborhood health centers have a higher proportion of people who have had no previous history of receiving mental health care than do other programs. The controversial hypothesis that location is more important than other factors in patients' decisions to use facilities could be tested by doing a replication of Stratmann's interesting study [17] within the research design.

Stratmann investigated the relative importance of various factors in patients' preferences for seeking health care at a given facility. The facilities studied were hospital emergency rooms, hospital outpatient departments, private physicians, work clinics, and neighborhood health centers. The factors influencing patients were grouped as economic (cost), temporal (hours of availability of service), convenience, sociopsychological (patient perception of staff qualities—honesty, courtesy, and so forth—not directly related to health care and service characteristics), and quality (patient's perception of staff and service characteristics directly related to health care—competence, correct diagnoses, appropriate referrals, and so forth). People were interviewed who were actually attending given facilities, and others drawn from the general population were asked which facilities they had chosen and would choose the next time they needed health care. Results showed differences in the ordering of preferences for patients at different facilities, and also that choice of facility and ordering of preferences varied by age, sex, income, and health status. Some principal findings were that people with low education and income, black, female, and/or Spanish-speaking, tended to stress the importance of sociopsychological factors in their choice of service, while richer, younger people listed these factors as *less* important than physical convenience or quality of care. If poorer people were in poor health, however, quality of care became as important as sociopsychological factors.

Similarly, many of the hypotheses concerning the complicated relationships between social class, utilization, and outcome, widely discussed in the mental health field [16], could be examined at least tentatively within this design.

In using this chapter as a basis for such theoretic research, the following advice may be helpful:

1. Be as clear as possible about the problems you are trying to solve and the questions you are trying to answer.
2. Conceptualize as many alternative hypotheses as you can which, if tested, might increase your understanding of these problems and questions.
3. Decide in advance as far as possible what criteria you will use for deciding whether the data obtained support or fail to support the hypotheses you choose to test. Some references provide more complex and detailed versions of this advice [23-25].

The following three sections indicate what data should be collected in order to provide as thorough an answer as possible to "What's going on here?" as well as a sound data base from which to attempt to generate criteria for judging what should be happening, to evaluate how closely the neighborhood health center in question is approximating the quality of service judged desirable, and to suggest where service might be improved.

The first section indicates the descriptive parametric data we suggest should be gathered. The second discusses some issues and possibilities concerning patient improvement and satisfaction measures. The third outlines how the study attempts to identify specific problems and strengths in the delivery of service (see Appendix 12A which provides the more detailed design plan for use as an actual blueprint for an evaluation. Specific data forms and protocols can be obtained from the authors.)

Description of Patients, Staff, and Services

Characteristics of Patients Served. This portion of the study identifies the patients served at each facility on a number of demographic, social, and psychological dimensions. It thus makes possible a description of the patient population served at each facility and also makes possible a comparison of facilities so that one can determine the differences, if any, between populations actually served at various facilities.

A. Demographic characteristics: age, sex, marital and parental status, composition of household, race, religion, address;

B. Socioeconomic characteristics (education, occupation, employment status, income);

C. Medical and psychiatric current diagnoses. These are recorded recognizing that there may well be differences between facilities in how and how often a diagnosis is actually made, and in how diagnostic categories are actually used. These problems make any comparison between facilities on this dimension extremely hazardous. Therefore, these data will be used primarily as a basis for generating questions about the different facilities. In the more intensive interview study of patients served at each facility it will be possible to make psychiatric diagnoses and symptom ratings by the research interviewer so that there will be possible meaningful comparisons of the psychiatric status of patients served at each facility.

D. Previous use of health care and mental health care facilities: number of recorded ambulatory visits and hospital days for all conditions in the year prior to the day the patient is counted for the study. Once again, validity of these figures for any one facility and for comparison between facilities depends on accurate records. These are not always kept in community facilities, and in any actual research setting the researchers will have to ascertain personally the extent to which records are or are not kept in each facility studied. Where data are not available, rough estimates based on the 50-patient intensive study may be made.

The number of representative patients served, compared to population from which they are drawn can only be ascertained for facilities which serve a defined population. As a practical matter, the defined population must have already been described by someone else since the expense of defining it for this study would be prohibitive. Therefore, in practical terms, we are dealing with geographically defined populations. Since the entire country is divided into census tracts and since for each tract considerable demographic and socioeconomic information is available from the Bureau of the Census, then if the facility serves any census tract or tracts in toto, it is possible to compare the patients served from that census area with the total population of the area and determine to what extent particular groups of people (for example, men, people over 65, people with less than a high school education, and so forth) are overutilizing or underutilizing the facility.

If two facilities serve the same census tract, for example, an emergency psychiatric service at a general hospital and a neighborhood health center, then a direct comparison of utilization rates for the two facilities becomes possible.

Since all neighborhood health centers serve defined areas, this portion of the study can be carried out at least for the NHC and possibly for other facilities as well.

Services Provided to Patients in the Five Facilities.

A. Types of patient care available (e.g., psychiatric evaluations; individual and group therapy; marriage, alcohol, drug counseling; consultation to other caregiving personnel; day care, home visiting; special programs for the elderly, children, adolescents, and so forth).

B. Hours of service (day, evening, night, emergency, or walk-in).

C. Staff (professional categories, paraprofessionals, years of experience, hours per week assigned to staff supervision and training).

D. How much service does each facility render and how many people does it serve? How many new patients come for service per unit time? How many return visits and distribution of visits per patient? How many broken appointments?

Consultation Services. The foregoing questions all relate to the delivery of direct mental health services as opposed to indirect or consultative services. One advantage of the NHC, as well as of the general hospital psychiatric service and of the health maintenance organization, is that each one offers the potential for close working relationships between mental health and primary health care professionals. Thus the opportunity exists for frequent and informal case consultation so that mental health expertise may have an impact on persons who do not actually receive direct mental health services. Therefore, we suggest a further category by which the five facilities may be compared:

How much case consultation is actually given by each facility? How much program consultation is given by each facility?

Improvement and Satisfaction of Patients

As part of the attempt to estimate whether the neighborhood health center being evaluated provides care at least equal in quality to that of other existing facilities we suggest addressing two questions:

A. Do patients improve or not after service is rendered?

B. Are patients satisfied or not with the service they receive?

(The specific measures we suggest for answering each of these are presented in Appendix 12A.) Again, collection of these data offers the opportunity for describing each facility individually and for comparing all of the facilities with each other.

This part of the study deals with three variables, quality of care, outcome of treatment, and patient satisfaction which are among the most notoriously difficult either to conceptualize or to measure in the mental health field. It has been said, for example, that goals of treatment differ from patient to patient. In one case, the goal may be curative and in another palliative. In some ways, the search for one measure of quality of care may be analogous to a search for the measure of the quality of life, illusive to say the least. Who can say what quality means for each person [10].

Outcome studies, it has been pointed out, are theoretically problematic [26, 27], time-consuming, and expensive. We agree, however, with Linn and Linn who note: "The fact that many problems exist in measuring outcome does not mean that measurement of outcome should not be attempted . . . other methods of evaluating care can only be a substitute." [10] These authors suggest that outcome should be measured multidimensionally with separate measurements made for an individual's social adjustment, level of physical and psychological symptoms and satisfaction, and then analyzed together using multivariate statistical techniques.

It is our impression, however, that the evaluator of a NHC's mental health services need not tackle all the dimensions and problems of measuring outcome, but should at least try to use some established, standardized measure of social adjustment and symptom level to measure baseline function and improvement rates in each facility, and then to make comparisons between patients in different facilities. The measures we suggest are not difficult to make; we do not suggest, however, that the analysis of them for the purposes of comparing facilities and evaluating a particular NHC will be anything but problematic. Just one difficult consideration is that the very population NHCs hope to serve is one suffering from the most intractable combinations of life problems and physical and psychological symptoms. It may be of value in itself that these people are in treatment at all. Still, an outcome study should be attempted as part of a thorough data base for evaluation.

Since outcome is so problematic a matter, we suggest separating this measure, both in concept and presentation, from the measure of patient satisfaction; the measure obtained, however, could be incorporated in a multivariate analysis of outcome as suggested above [23]. It has been noted that "the role of patient satisfaction remains a topic barely examined by health researchers" [28] and that techniques to measure it "are still somewhat primitive" [10]. Still, we have suggested some questions (Appendix 12A) which attempt not just to provide global measures of satisfaction but also information on what people have liked or disliked about their mental health services.

Problems in Quality of Service Delivery

Although evidence that problems exist may be derived from the descriptive, outcome, and satisfaction measures already referred to, a precise account of problems can only be made by careful observation of the facility at work. The three-part, interfacility, comparative study protocol presented here provides a particularly good tool for locating, analyzing, and suggesting solutions to problems. Becoming familiar with patients and staff during Parts Two and Three of the study (Appendix 12A) would enable the evaluator to observe, follow up cases, and hear a variety of opinions about the difficulties of obtaining or providing service in the facility that is rarely obtained by means of questionnaires alone [29]. Furthermore, when a problem has been identified in the facility to be evaluated, the researcher has the opportunity of asking him or herself why it does not occur in the other facilities observed. The answer may well suggest the solution, or limitations of proposed solutions in the NHC under study.

Summary

This chapter and appendices present a protocol for a research project which we believe can be carried out in any of a variety of facilities that deliver ambulatory psychiatric services. We have tried to present the plan with sufficient generality so that it can be applied in any facility of one's choice, and, at the same time, we have tried to present the method with sufficient specificity so that a reader can actually carry out the project if he so desires.

The method can be used to test a variety of hypotheses related to service delivery. To consider only one of current interest, there is considerable concern at the moment regarding the community treatment of deinstitutionalized former mental hospital patients. The question has been raised repeatedly as to what followup, if any, many of these discharged patients are receiving. We might hypothesize that former state hospital patients are more likely to receive care in a neighborhood health center than in a general hospital psychiatric outpatient service. From the data obtained from Part One of Appendix 12A, such patients could be identified, and the proportion of such patients among the various facilities under study could be determined.

If one wished to study these patients more intensively one could study the experience of consecutive former state hospital patients seeking service at one or more ambulatory treatment facilities using the method outlined in Part Two (Appendix 12A). One would then be able to learn something about treatment results and short-term outcome as well as about utilization. Similarly, the method can be applied to any other definable group of patients in which there is theoretical interest or particular clinical concern.

Conclusion

Evaluation research is a life crisis for a mental health facility, but it is one which,

like other life crises, offers the potential for growth. It is the task of the researchers not only to carry out the research but to work with the professional staff so
that the fears related to evaluation can be adequately explored and dealt with and
so that the experience is one which leads to crisis resolution and growth. If this
is done, the facility staff will be free to examine their experience with the research
staff in a way which most professionals rarely have the opportunity to do. Talking about what has gone right as well as what has gone wrong makes it possible
to question one's assumptions and to seek additional training and supervision to
help with one's weaknesses. Obviously the administrator of the facility must be
aware of this aspect of the research experience and be prepared to support his
staff as the results are shared. If this is done, and if the work is published or
otherwise communicated publicly, gains for the professional world outside the
facility are in addition to those which accrue to the staff of the facility, patients
and potential patients, and the neighborhood.

Appendix 12A

Design and Method for a Comparison of a Neighborhood Health Center Providing Mental Health Services and Other Low-Cost Mental Health Services

Below are listed the steps suggested for conducting a three-part evaluation study of five different mental health services. We will not repeat here the facilities which could be compared or the basic questions which the data collected should be used to answer. There will be no further suggestions for analysis of the data, although clearly the possibilities are legion. (Specific data forms and protocols may be obtained from the authors.)

Part One — Description of Patients, Staff and Services

Obtain information on:

1. All types of mental health service offered.
2. Hours of operation of each service.
3. Number of patients seen per month at each service:
   a. new visits;
   b. return visits;
   c. broken appointments.
4. Number of staff and number of hours involved in:
   a. direct patient care;
   b. consultation;
   c. supervision and teaching
5. Patient data as follows (on at least 100 consecutive different patients at each facility): age, sex, marital status, number of children, age of oldest and youngest child, occupation, years of education, weekly income (averaged for past month), ethnic group, main language, medical problems requiring current treatment or medication, previous use of mental health services, referral pathway to facility, contacts with other social agencies and health care providers within the last 30 days.

This information may be obtained in various ways. If facility routinely collects such information and it is available for processing, it may easily be obtained (if so, it may be equally possible, and preferrable, to collect the patient information for a year). The service and staff data may be obtained from descriptive brochures and annual reports providing the researcher has checked the accuracy of these with appropriate personnel. Other methods include the design of a questionnaire to be filled in by staff members on each of 100 consecutive patients seen or by the researcher working with office and treatment staff. Where information (e.g., previous use of mental health services) proves impossible to obtain except by direct contact with the patient, the results of Part Two should be used.

Part Two — Improvement and Satisfaction of Patients

In each facility, a defined sample of 50 patients should be studied by interview and observation. It is desirable that the entire study be done by two observers, although only one researcher will observe any one interview or staff member. Two observers is the appropriate number for the following considerations: if there is only one interviewer, there is no possibility of establishing inter-rater reliability on those instruments for which it is possible to establish such reliability. It is important that every interviewer do an equal number of interviews at each facility so that interviewer and facility are not confounded. If this study is to be successful, the interviewers must have good working relations with the facility staff. The larger the number of interviewers, the more difficult it is to establish those working relationships. Hence, two research interviewers is the optimum number. The work could be done by only one interviewer, but he or she would have to establish reliability with some second person in any case. Another disadvantage of using only one interviewer is that the study would require an unreasonable length of time to complete.

Sample Selection

It is important not to confound order of interviewing with facility; that is, one should not simply interview 50 consecutive patient/clients in one facility and then move on to the next facility, since it may well be that the interviewer's technique will change over time. It is necessary, therefore, to do some portion of the 50 in each of the five facilities and then do the remaining portions in a counterbalanced order [25].

Method

Prior to the start of the study, the study staff must obtain informed consent for the study from the governing board or other administratively responsible body for each facility, and must then work with the staff to obtain their informed consent, and finally must obtain from each individual person served his or her informed consent to participate in the study.

Informed consent is of critical importance to the success of this or any similar study. Not only persons served but staff of neighborhood health centers as well as governing boards are uniquely sensitive to the possible exploitation of patients. For this reason, Appendix 12B includes our proposed informed consent form. (Forms to record all other data are available on request from the authors.)

For each 50 patients studied intensively in each facility, the social and psychiatric data in the questionnaire should be obtained. In addition, three interviews should be conducted to ascertain the treatment experience of each patient, and to gather other basic data on overall level of functioning, symptoms, and specific problems of social functioning.

Notes on First Interview

1. The initial visit of patients to any mental health service of each of the facilities should be observed. As soon as possible after the initial clinical interviews, the researcher should complete his or her report. Immediately, if possible, following the initial service interview, the researcher should interview the patient in order to make the following ratings:

a. Complete a standard symptom rating scale. We suggest the Hopkins Symptom checklist [30], to be completed by the patient with the interviewer's help.

b. Rate the patient's overall level of psychological functioning using the Menninger Health-Sickness Rating Scale. This scale is used to rate each person on a scale which spans the whole range of psychiatric disability and personal functioning [31]. One hundred represents a healthy, happy person; zero represents a person institutionalized, psychotic, and unable to care for himself. (It should be possible to make this rating, at least roughly, based on the clinical interview alone, in most cases.)

c. Rate the patient's level of social functioning, using one of two instruments. For people at the sicker end of the health-sickness scale, i.e., below 50, the researcher should use the Strauss-Carpenter social functioning scale which has been developed for use with schizophrenic patients [33].

For patients scoring above 60, the researcher should use selected items from Gurland's Structured and Scaled Interview to Assess Maladjustment [32] as follows: the complete interview focuses on five problem areas: work, social-leisure, family of origin, marriage, and sex. If the patient has complained of problems in one or two of these areas, the researcher should ask the questions relating to those areas. No more than two areas should be covered because to do so would require so much of the patient's time that the research interview would begin to loom larger in his or her experience at the facility than the clinical interview. In other words, the act of measurement would change the experience to such an extent as to interfere seriously with what we are trying to study.

For patients scoring between 50 and 60 on the health-sickness scale, the

researcher should complete the Strauss-Carpenter Scale and one problem area
from the Gurland. For patients complaining of no problem area from the Gurland
but scoring above 60, complete the Strauss-Carpenter Scale (few such patients
exist). At the conclusion of the interview, make a final health-sickness rating.

2. One month after the initial visit the staff member who saw the patient
first should be interviewed by the researcher to ascertain the facts of the patient's
history in the facility subsequent to the first interview. Assessment should also
be made of the staff person's level of knowledge about the patient.

3. Three months after the initial visit the researcher should re-interview the
patient about his/her treatment experience, status of the difficulties initially
present and present ones, and re-assess the symptoms and social functioning
using the initial procedures again. At this time the patient's opinion about the
service received should be obtained with a view to estimating overall satisfaction.
We suggest first asking open-ended questions about what was experienced as
most and least helpful about the patient's contacts with the facility, and later
asking specifically about cost, time, location, staff courteousness and competence,
helpfulness with the patient's problem, and willingness of the patient to return
or recommend the facility to a friend. Forms devised by the authors also indicate the wording and order in which questions should be asked, a matter of
crucial importance in obtaining comparable satisfaction ratings.

Notes on Second Interview

If the evaluation is completed in one session, i.e., if the clinician does not plan to
see the patient again, the interview with the clinician may be conducted immediately and data forms completed. If the patient is seen more than once by
the initial clinician, this form may be completed any time after the first interview,
up to but not longer than one month.

Researcher should organize his or her impressions of staff person's understanding of patient's needs and difficulties. In addition to the treatment history,
a checklist should be made of items to be learned by a mental health staff person
during the first few interviews with a new patient. The authors' forms provide a
possible protocol, but a new one may be necessary after the researcher has consulted with experienced supervisory personnel at the facilities to be evaluated and
observed a number of patient interviews on a pre-test basis.

Notes on Third Interview

Three months after the initial observed interview, the researcher should reinterview
the patient, which should include reestimation of all the symptom and functioning
ratings initially made. It is particularly important in these interviews to note

verbatim statements about the patient's experience in the facility attended and views about the way in which he or she was treated, helped, the mode of referral, and so forth. Patients should be interviewed in a setting most comfortable and convenient for them, for example, before or after a clinic visit, at their home, in a local bar or restaurant. Experience with follow-up interviews of this kind has led to the conclusion that most patients welcome the opportunity to discuss themselves and their treatment, and consider it more an example of being noticed and cared for than an intrusion. Some effort must be made to assure them that negative as well as positive comments about the facility are being sought, and that no blame is being attached if the patient has not followed through with a treatment plan.

Part Three — Problems in Quality of Service Delivery

Part Three is designed to establish (1) the amount of consultation rendered in each of these five facilities; (2) whether differences exist in how staff spend their time in different facilities; (3) problems in service delivery as perceived by staff. The method of this study is participant observation; the researcher should "shadow" one staff member for a three-day period of time. The researcher should not shadow the staff member continuously, but up to the point at which a clinical service is rendered in private to a patient or client. The researcher will resume shadowing him when he has completed the service. In this way the confidentiality of the staff-patient contact will be preserved but the researcher will have an opportunity to observe all staff-staff interactions, and monitor all phone calls except those that occur during patient service episodes. The person shadowed will be asked to record each interaction—who is spoken with, the general subject, and the outcome of the call.

For each interpersonal contact during the day the researcher will record name and status of the contact, subject discussed, outcome of discussion, i.e., action recommended or taken, and time elapsed.

At each facility, observations should be made on two psychiatrists, two other mental health professionals, and to mental health workers, each for a three-day period. If the facility has only one staff member in one of these categories, then only one will be observed. If the facility does not have full-time staff in any category, each staff person will be observed for a minimum of ten hours, however many working days that requires, and the staff member will also be interviewed about work problems. Staff to be observed will be selected randomly from among all staff, of the appropriate category, who have worked in the facility for a least one year. If there are no staff in any category who have worked for one year or more, then the two staff who have worked longest and have membership in the appropriate category will be selected.

In order for all three parts of the study to be carried out, it will be necessary for the researcher(s) to become familiar with the staff of the various facilities, and for the staff to become familiar with them and trust them sufficiently to permit the study to be performed. Obviously the choice of research interviewers is critical to the success of such studies. The person must have not only the independence of a research person and the training and skills to conduct interviews in an unbiased manner, but must also have sufficient warmth and interest in other human beings to communicate a genuine concern for the staff and their endeavors. Again, if this is not communicated, the presence of the researchers is likely to lead to such discomfort and resentment as to interfere with the clinical services in a way that will render the research meaningless.

Appendix 12B

Patient Consent Form

At the present time some of the staff of this facility, in collaboration with some independent mental health professionals, are attempting to evaluate the service rendered by this facility. The aims of the study are to describe the people served by this facility as compared to other facilities, to describe the services offered to the people who come here, and to find out what happens to the people who come here over a three-month period. For example, if they come with a problem, is it better, the same, or worse? Did the person feel he was helped, was not helped, or was worse off as a result of coming to the facility?

This is what we are asking of you. We want to have an independent observer sit in during your first interview. This observer will also interview you at your convenience—either right after your interview here today or sometime in the next day or two at a time and place of your choosing. In three months the interviewer will contact you for one last interview to find out how you are doing at that time. All of the information we obtain will be entirely confidential. We will not release any information about any patient to anyone in this study, nor will we discuss our findings with anyone except, if you give your permission, with the staff here, but only if they and you both want us to.

We may, as a result of this research, prepare a paper which will be used to help the facility justify its present budget and/or obtain additional funds. We may also share our findings about the facility and group of patients with the larger professional community if we think this would be of value. We will not, in any published writing, publish any data which permit identification of any person who participates in this study.

Your participation in this study is entirely voluntary. You will receive exactly the same service here whether or not you agree to participate in this research. The advantage to you in participating is not large; perhaps it will help the facility and hence indirectly help you; perhaps the additional research interviews will be helpful to you or to the staff here in understanding you better. However, we are certain that the research will not hurt you in any way, and it is possible that the research project will be socially useful. We hope that you will agree to participate. Copies of all written research reports will be available at the facility and will be given to any participant who wants one.

References

1. Donabedian A. Evaluating the Quality of Mental Health Care. *Milbank Memorial Fund Quarterly* XLIV (part 2), 166-206, 1966.

2. Zussman J., Slawson M. Service Quality Profile, Development of a Technique for Measuring Quality of Mental Health Services. *Arch Gen. Psych.* 27: 692-98, 1972.

3. Fox P.D. Some Approaches to Evaluating Community Mental Health Services. *Arch. Gen. Psych.* 20: 172-8, 1972.

4. Zussman, J. and Reiff E.R. Evaluation of the Quality of Mental Health Services. *Arch. Gen. Psych* 20: 352-357, 1969.

5. Beck, J.C. "Record Keeping and Research," in *The Practice of Community Mental Health*, Grunebaum, H., Ed. Boston: Little Brown, 1970.

6. Rappaport M. Evaluating Community Health Services: Guidelines for an Administrator. *Hosp. Commun. Psych.* 24: 757-60, 1973.

7. Lombillo J., Kiresuk, T.J., and Sherman, R.E. Evaluating a Community Mental Health Program: Contract Fulfillment Analysis. *Hosp. Commun. Psych.* 24: 760-2, 1973.

8. Glotz B., Rusk, T.N., and Sternbach, R.S. A Built-In Evaluation System in a New Community Mental Health Program. *Am. J. Publ. Health* 63: 702-9, 1973.

9. Miller S.I., and Schlachter, R.H. A Multidimensional Problem-Oriented Review and Evaluation System. *Am. J. Psych.* 132: 232-5, 1975.

10. Linn, M.W. and Linn, B.S. Narrowing the Gap Between Medical and Mental Health Evaluation, *Medical Care*, 13: 607-614, 1975.

11. Landsberg, G. and Taylor, S. Evaluating a Center's Multiservice Program for the Self-Sufficient Elderly. *Hosp. Commun. Psych.* 24: 557-60, 1973.

12. Lowe, E.D. and Alston, J.P. An Analysis of Racial Differences in Service to Alcoholics in a Southern Clinic. *Hosp. Commun. Psych.* 24: 547-50, 1973.

13. Fox, R. and Potter, N.D. Using Inpatient Staff for Aftercare of Severely Disturbed Chronic Patients. *Hosp. Commun. Psych.* 24: 482-4, 1973.

14. Wing, J.K. and Hailey, A.M. *Evaluating a Community Psychiatric Service.* London: Oxford University Press, 1972.

15. Collver, A., et al., Factors Influencing the Use of Maternal Health Services. *Soc. Sci and Med.* 1: 293-308, 1967.

16. McKinlay, J. Some Approaches and Problems in the Study of the Use of Services. *J. of Health and Soc. Behav.* 13: 115-152, 1972.

17. Stratmann, W.C. A Study of Consumer Attitudes about Health Care: The Delivery of Ambulatory Services. *Medical Care,* 13: 537-548, 1975.

18. Sparer, G., Anderson, A. Cost of Services at Neighborhood Health Centers. *New Eng. J. Med.* 286: 1241-45, 1972.

19. Cooper, E. Myles. *Guidelines for a Minimum Statistical and Accounting System for Community Mental Health Centers.* U.S. Dept. of Health, Education, and Welfare; Alcohol, Drug Abuse, and Mental Health Administration. DHEW Publication Number HSM 42-72-194 (1973).

20. Feldman, S. and Windle, C. The NIMH Approach to Evaluating the Community Mental Health Center Programs. *Health Services Reports* Vol. 88 No. 2 (February, 1973).

21. Sorenson, J.E. and Phipps, D.W. Cost Finding: A tool for Managing your Community Mental Health Center, Administration in Mental Health. U.S. Dept. of Health, Education, and Welfare, National Institute of Mental Health. DHEW Pub. No. (HSM) 73-9050, Winter, 1972.

22. Menn, Hubert L. Developing Principles of Cost Finding for Community Mental Health Centers. *Am. J. of Pub. Health.* Vol. 61 No. 8, August, 1971.

23. Overall, J.E. and Klett, C.J. *Applied Multivariate Analysis.* New York: McGraw-Hill, 1972.

24. Miller, D.C. *Handbook of Research Design and Social Measurement.* New York: David McKay, 1964.

25. Hyman, H. *Survey Design and Analysis.* Glencoe, Ill.: Free Press, 1955.

26. Malan, D. The Outcome Problem in Psychotherapy: Research. *Arch. Gen. Psychiat.* 29: 719-729, 1973.

27. Mintz, J: What is Success in Psychotherapy? *J. Abnor. Psychology* 80: 11-19, 1972.

28. Fink, R.: The Measurement of Medical Care Utilization, in Greenlick, R. *Conceptual Issues in the Analysis of Medical Care Utilization Behavior.* Dept. of Health Education and Welfare, Public Health Serv: 5, 1970.

29. Lebow, J.L. Consumer Assessments of the Quality of Medical Care. *Medical Care,* 12: 328, 1974.

30. Derogatis, L.R., et al. The Hopkins Symptom Checklist: A Measure of Primary Symptom Dimensions. In *Psychological Measurements in Psychopharmacology: Modern Problems in Pharmopsychiatry,* Pichot, P., Ed. Vol 7 S Kargel, Basel Switzerland, 1974.

31. Luborsky L., The Health-Sickness Rating Scale, *Bull. Menninger Clinic* 39: 448-480, 1975.

32. Gurland, B.J., et al. The Structured and Scaled Interview to Assess Maladjustment (SSIAM). *Arch. Gen. Psych.* 27: 259-267, 1972.

33. Strauss, J.S. and Carpenter, W.T. The Prediction of Outcome in Schizophrenia *Arch. Gen. Psych.* 27: 739-746, 1972.

34. Luborsky, L. and Backrach, H. Factors Influencing Clinician's Judgments of Mental Health. *Arch. Gen. Psych.* 31, 1974, 292-299.

13

Evaluation of Neighborhood Mental Health Centers

Robert L. Leopold and Richard D. Kluft

One of the new institutions of the community mental health center movement [1], whose emergence was also related to simultaneous social and political
changes, has been the small outpatient treatment center described variously as
the satellite clinic, storefront clinic, crisis center, or neighborhood center. These
units, regardless of label, are outpatient facilities in an overall system providing
in its totality the basic, federally mandated mental health services. Despite the
diverse forms they have assumed, they differ from other community mental
health care delivery channels in being relatively free standing and located within
the population area to which they are mandated providers of mental health care.
These characteristics result in arrangements different from those in other facilities
and contexts, such as: a central facility (often a state hospital) staffed by teams,
each responsible for a separate catchment area; situations in which a part of a
general medical center (such as a large hospital) is designated as a CMHC; and
circumstances in which an agency contracts out to numerous preexisting facilities
and/or practitioners for provision of basic services. These units, hereafter referred
to as neighborhood or local clinics, have a considerable but variable degree of
autonomy. Most often they assume a form dictated by considerations of community needs and priorities and staff preferences and capabilities.

Initially, the establishment of such centers stemmed from the wish to treat
the mentally ill person in his own community in order to avoid the difficulties,
complications, and expense inherent in reliance upon the state hospital systems.
It was felt that a small and unobtrusive unit, located among its service consumers,
would be more accessible, less foreign and imposing, and less stigmatizing to
both the individual client-patient and the overall community than a large central
edifice. It was hoped that as the unit developed ties with the community it
served, its relation to its community would improve, and consultation, education,
and preventive services would be facilitated. In many cases, plans to develop
community residents as indigenous therapists have been implemented as part of
this trend.

In the process of working in their communities, such centers have often contributed significantly to community well being. Unfortunately, in addition,
often they have become involved, by unquestioningly accepting community

The authors wish to thank Elias S. Cohen, M.P.A., J.D., Project Director; Edith A. Leopold,
Ph.D., and Lawrence Schein, B.A., Research Directors, for making their data available to us.

community priorities as their own, in activities beyond their capacity and skill, and have suffered diffusion and frustration [2].

A variety of arguments have been advanced on behalf of the local health center. All of these can be reduced to the attempt to answer affirmatively one basic question: Can the neighborhood center make a more relevant total response to the idiosyncratic needs and wishes of the community it serves than a more centralized point of delivery? To this must be added a subsidiary, but vitally important, question: Can it do so on a cost-effective basis? What emerges, however, as one of the least emotion-laden but most significant problem areas in this issue is the difficulty the small center experiences in arranging for the overall treatment of its patients/clients. The multiproblem consumer is the rule rather than the exception on many center caseloads, and is a challenge to the ability of the center to manage itself as a portal vis-à-vis the whole system of human services. Many of the local center's strengths reside in its autonomy and local orientation, but these assets can rapidly become liabilities to many patients/clients. Although the center is a portal, an entryway, into the totality of health and human service care, it in itself is so small that its multiple-problem patients/clients almost inevitably face a built-in fragmentation of care. The overall facilitation of patient care is inherently complicated for the local center by the need to manage communications and linkages with other branches of the same system, and also with other systems. The demand for an overall comprehensive outlook thus clashes at crucial junctures with the virtues inherent in the local center's basic orientation.

As in all planning endeavors, certain structural difficulties of the local center were overlooked. Because of the small staff, continuity of care and comprehensive response to patient needs cannot be rendered solely by local centers in all cases; neighborhood linkages with community resources are sometimes rendered inoperative by decisions made at distant points. The total pool of staff available is diluted, so that each local clinic may offer a weaker clinical program than the total staff could provide if united geographically. Moreover, each staff member must play multiple roles, some of which are uncomfortable or unknown to him. Perhaps the greatest potential problem in the neighborhood center lies in the area of program development; because the staff is small, adequate program preparation time is scarce. Further, the center's necessary and desirable involvement with the community can lead to a felt need to respond to multiple and conflicting requests, some of which are irrational, some inappropriate, and some unattainable, given available resources. If the local staff needs to negotiate with its parent agency for planning help, it finds it must give up valuable clinical or outreach time to do so. Many centers have been plunged into areas where they lack impact and ability and come away with bitter disappointment in their efforts and with marked community disenchantment.

Background of Current Study

Despite an almost magical belief in the efficacy of neighborhood delivery of mental health services, few studies present substantial objective data which evaluate the performance of the local mental health centers. Fewer still have done so in terms of centers' responsiveness to the independently assessed overall needs of their consumer constituency. In view of this, this chapter presents data derived from a recently completed study of the Department of Community Medicine of the University of Pennsylvania. The data which follow are drawn from this study, and we are indebted to the investigators for making it available freely to us. The study was conducted in part at the 43rd Street Counseling Center, one of seven such centers of the West Philadelphia Community Mental Health Consortium. (Details concerning the founding, administration, and program of the Consortium are available elsewhere [3]). To recapitulate briefly, the Consortium, a federally funded community mental health center, has a catchment area in West Philadelphia of just over 200,000 persons. The Consortium was designed from the start as a decentralized operation, with decentralization occurring at or near the geographical locations of its member hospitals. Within the first few months of operation, local mental health centers were established in the belief that these decentralized centers could accommodate more easily to local differences than could larger units. Each local center operates with overall administrative guidance from the Consortium and with ongoing supervision.

The 43rd Street Counseling Center serves a subcatchment area of approximately 40,000 people, and is housed in the same facility as the Philadelphia Health Department District Office. Over the past four years (for which figures are available), it has consistently been the largest provider of services among the Consortium's counseling centers and performed 28 percent of all interviews conducted at counseling centers. It was thus seen as presenting an unusual opportunity to forge linkages between the local delivery of mental health services and the local delivery of general preventive health services provided by the Public Health Center, particularly since these two units occupied the same building. (Table 13-1 presents titles and functions of the 43rd Street staff.)

The full-time staff of eight consists of six engaged in direct patient treatment—the center director, chief social worker, two additional social workers, an alcoholism counselor, and a mental health assistant; a registrar and secretary-receptionist provide administrative assistance. The part-time people are: the staff psychiatrist, who consults with staff, participates in case conferences, prescribes and reviews medications, and leads one socialization group for chronic patients; a psychiatrist specializing in family therapy; a psychiatrist advising on school and community consultation from the Consortium's Consultation, Education, and Training Department; a generalist physician from the Alcoholism program who tends to the medication needs of alcoholic patients and provides physical examinations when necessary; a caseworker from a child guidance center; and a social work student on field placement.

The administrative function resides in the director. The supervision of ongoing treatment is the responsibility of the chief social worker and the psychiatrist, with special assistance from the director,

Table 13-1.
Titles and Functions of 43rd Street Staff

Titles	Admin- istration	Direct Supervision	Consul- tation	General Patient Care	Special Patient Care	School Consul- tation	General Medicine	Pharmaco- therapy	Non- Treatment
Full Time:									
Director	+	+				+			
Chief Social Worker		+		+					
Social Worker				+					
Social Worker				+					
Mental Health Assistant				+					
Alcoholism Counselor					+				
Secretary-Receptionist									+
Registrar									+
Part Time:									
Staff Psychiatrist		+	+	+				+	
Family Therapist			+						
School Consult/Psychiatrist			+			+			
Student Social Worker				+					
General Physician					+		+	+	
Child Guidance Worker				+					
Totals	1	3	3	8	2	2	1	2	2

a supervisor to whom the alcoholism worker reports, and from the family therapist.

The Health Network Project (HNP) was designed to evaluate the entrance of patients and clients into the health and welfare system through four portals in West Philadelphia. Thus, only a low-income population was studied. The entry points studied were: the District Public Assistance Office, the Child Welfare Office, the Emergency Room of a general hospital, and the 43rd Street Center. Attempts were made to identify presenting problems, the response to these problems, and particularly the linkages both within and outside the portals studied, to determine the effectiveness or ineffectiveness of client flow through a linked system of care.

Methodology

The initial sampling design called for both prospective and retrospective interviews of 125 financially eligible, newly and consecutively registered patients. This comprised about 25 percent of projected annual registrants and provided an appreciation of the patient's presenting circumstances and his appraisal of the agency after several sessions of therapy. Complications and time restrictions emerged, necessitating modifications. Because a previously approved ongoing study rendered incoming patients largely inaccessible, three retrospective groups were tapped to gain sufficient single interviews for the study-registrants for two calendar periods in addition to a random selection from current caseloads. The sample population was therefore neither consecutive nor anterospective.

Nearly one fourth of the center's patients were above study limits in terms of income. However, the 87 patients interviewed comprised 28 percent of the 310 whose records were consulted; 36 of the 237 eligibles could not be interviewed before the study ended, and 5 patients, under 3 percent of the eligibles, refused to be interviewed. Those interviewed were paid $10 for their participation. They were seen at the center (24 or 28 percent), the Department of Community Medicine (37 or 42 percent), or in their homes (26 or 30 percent).

Selected Data

The demographic characteristics of 43rd Street Center patients and their households are summarized in Summary Table 13-2. At least one prior attempt to obtain treatment was made by 77 percent of the patients before coming to the Counseling Center—two thirds of these by going to hospitals. Indeed, nearly one half of the patients seen at 43rd Street were referred *from* hospital units. However, the referral pattern was by no means clear, and often the visit to the hospital must be viewed an an antecedent contact and not as a clearcut referral.

Table 13-2

Selected Interportal Data for Health Network Project Samples of Clients/Patients and Households

Demographic and Socioeconomic Characteristics

(All figures are *percents* unless otherwise noted)

| | Portal | | | | |
Item	Receiving Ward	CBA-West	43rd Street	Child Welfare	All Portals
Median age of clients/pts. (yrs)	20.8	32.2	29.4	10.6[a]	—
Households with children present	67.8	71.6	34.5	90.2	68.7
Population per household	4.36	4.12	3.19	4.33	4.11
Households with unrelated persons	12.6	17.3	40.2	9.8	17.7
Tenant households	88.9	64.9	77.4	NA[b]	—
Less than 2 yrs at present address	44.6	53.8	57.5	NA	—
Welfare recipients among clients	83.3	100.0	61.6	64.2	80.0
Unemployed client/pt. labor force[c]	60.5	92.9	61.7	NA	—
Households with no one employed	74.0	74.6	51.9	55.0	63.8
Ill health as job problem for those those interested in work	53.0	25.0	37.1	NA	—
Median monthly household income	$269	$245	$211	NA	—
Welfare as *sole* source of household income	57.6	57.0	40.2	47.7	52.5

Source: Health Network Project, Department of Community Medicine, University of Pennsylvania, School of Medicine, 1971.

[a]Median age of the population of 122 mothers and 216 index children.

[b]NA-Not Available.

[c]Base for percent is the adult labor force combining full and part time employed persons with unemployed persons.

In terms of the hypothesis that a local center can provide optimal continuity of care, it is instructive to look at the outcome data: 26 of 87 patients interviewed were no longer in treatment; 12 were terminated by the agency; 14 were dropouts and still registered (the study data does not provide adequate information as to whether attempts to follow up patients were unsuccessful). Fifty-nine percent of patients reported having attended the clinic for three to nine months, and the frequency of treatment varied; 43 percent were seen once a week, and 30 percent were seen every two weeks.

The presenting problems were classified as indicated on Table 13-3. Of the patients in the study, 85 percent received individual counseling, 60 percent

Table 13-3

Presenting Problem of 43rd Street Center Patients by Detailed Classification (American Psychiatric Association code applied to interview data)[a]

Classification	Patients	
Medical Conditions, Symptoms	Number	Percent
Diseases of Central Nervous System & Diseases of Nerves	2	2.4
Psychiatric Conditions, Symptoms		
Disturbances of Behavior		
Alcoholic Addiction, Alcoholism, Drunkenness	8	9.4
Anger(extreme), Aggressivity or Destructiveness	4	4.7
Drug Addiction (including narcotic overdose)	2	2.4
Marital Adjustment Problems	8	9.4
Suicide: Thoughts, Threats, and Attempts	5	5.9
Other Behavior Disturbances	7	8.2
Disturbances of Thought	4	4.7
Distrubances of Affect		
Anxiety, Fear or Panic	7	8.2
Depression	6	7.0
Other Categories		
"Nerves"	7	8.2
Personality Disorders and Neuroses	2	2.4
Psychoses	2	2.4
Mental Retardation	2	2.4
Ill-defined Mental/Emotional Conditions/Symptoms	19	22.3
Total	85	100.0
Broad Classification		
Specific Medical Conditions, Symptoms	2	2.4
Psychiatric Conditions/Symptoms	(83)	(97.6)
Disturbances of Behavior	34	40.0
Disturbances of Thought	4	4.7
Disturbances of Affect	13	15.3
Other Categories	13	15.3
Ill-Defined Conditions/Symptoms	19	22.3
Total	85	100.0
Unknown	2	

Source: Health Network Project, Department of Community Medicine, University of Pennsylvania School of Medicine—Sample, 43rd Street Counseling Center, 1971.

[a] American Psychiatric Association, *Diagnostic and Statistical Manual of Mental Disorders, Third Edition (DSM-11)*, 1968.

received medication either alone or with counseling, 20 percent were in family therapy, and more than one half of all were involved in a multiplicity of treatment modalities. At interview, 84.7 percent stated they were improved, 4.7 percent worse, and 10.6 percent the same. Despite this, and despite 90 percent being favorably impressed with their treatment, when rating their problems' severity, only 13.6 percent of the interviewees said they now had no problems and 32.1 percent said that their problems were slight. Therefore, favorable "reviews" do not necessarily imply the resolution of problems for a majority of patients. This casts light on a need to assess this phenomenon further. Do these findings, for example, suggest that problems prove to be chronic, or that treatment is of limited effectiveness or attractiveness, or that many dropped out before gaining the complete benefits that treatment might afford? This study provides no answers. Of the people with problems the agency did not entirely resolve, 22 were involved in entries into further portals. Formal referral involved 15.7 percent who sought additional aid via self-initiated processes (Figure 13-1). The study does not indicate the degree of success of these endeavors.

One of the most significant spinoffs of this study concerned the assessment of current health problems. Of patients entering the 43rd Street portal, slightly over one third reported one condition, medical or psychiatric, in addition to the index emotional problem. One fifth indicated as many as two or more current health problems. In essence, 55 percent indicated the presence of multiple health difficulties at the time of the interview (Table 13-4).

The nature of the patients' problems is indicated by Figure 13-2, which includes current and the most recently treated difficulties (within the last year), as well as a "grand total." Surprisingly, despite the youth of the population (median age 29.1 years), circulatory disease accounted for 18 percent of current health problems; and despite the patients' portal, under one fifth of the total illnesses were psychiatric. Table 13-5 indicates the extent of other problems encountered as well as staff assessment and referrals.

Perhaps more surprising still is the chronic nature of the problems encountered (Tables 13-6 and 13-7); almost 60 percent of current conditions persisted for over a year. Slightly over 37 percent of current problems, exclusive of the presenting complaint, had an onset five years or more prior to the interview. Of 72 other current health problems (not presenting complaint) in the sample, over four fifths had had recent attention or were under treatment. Furthermore, of households with more than one person (55 of 87 households), 14.5 percent contained other members with medical problems, 9 percent contained members with psychiatric problems, and another 14.5 percent had members with *both* types of problems. The picture that emerges is of a population with clusters of difficulties as opposed to single problems, and a population with a vast spectrum of chronic health and social service needs, most of which are beyond the direct scope of the 43rd Street Clinic.

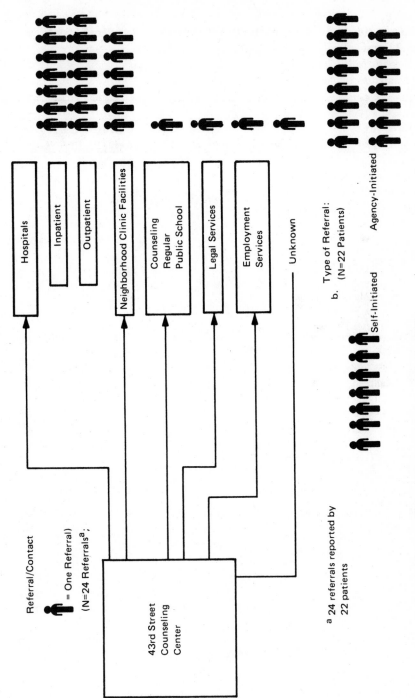

Source: Health Network Project Sample, 43rd Street Counseling Center, 1971.

[a]24 referrals reported by 22 patients.

Figure 13-1. Referrals from 43rd Street Counseling Center during treatment or at time of termination and type of referral.

Table 13-4

Selected Interportal Data for Health Network Project Samples of Clients/Patients and Households

Current Health Status

(All figures are *percents*)

	Portal				
Item	*Receiving Ward*	*CBA-West*	*43rd Street*	*Child Welfare[a]*	*All Portals*
Current health status inclusive of presenting problem[b]					
Clients/pts with one or more health problems	100.0	58.3	100.0	59.3	76.8
Clients/patients with multiple conditions	61.9	28.0	55.2	NA	–
Current health status exclusive of presenting problem[c]					
Clients/pts with medical problem(s)	49.7	50.8	43.6	56.0	51.3
Clients/pts with multiple medical conditions	21.0	20.2	17.2	22.7	20.9
Clients/pts with one or more psychiatric problems	34.8	26.1	13.7[d]	11.6[e]	13.5
Psychiatric conditions of all *conditions* reported	30.8	22.4	18.0	16.4	22.5
Conditions over 5 years duration	36.8	36.9	37.3	NA	–
Conditions untreated/no recent treatment	36.3	51.9	18.6	16.8	30.7
Conditions treated at hospitals	74.2	47.4	64.4	61.2	62.4
No regular contact with physician or dentist	47.0	50.8	51.7	NA	–
Major health problems among household members					
One or more major problems	44.0	51.7	38.1	71.1	52.4
Medical only	22.6	42.5	14.5	27.9	28.0
Psychiatric only	10.7	1.3	9.1	22.1	11.1
Medical *and* psychiatric	10.7	7.9	14.5	21.3	13.3

Source: Health Network Project, Department of Community Medicine, University of Pennsylvania School of Medicine, 1971.

[a]Except for the item on health of household members all Child Welfare health data refer to *index children.*

[b]The presenting problem for *all* patients at the Receiving Ward and at 43rd St. Counseling Center was a health problem. Patients at these portals with multiple health problems thus had one or more current health problems in addition to the presenting problem.

[c]Excludes the presenting health problem at Receiving Ward and 43rd St. Data for patients at these portals refer to current health conditions *other* than the presenting problem.

Table 13-4 — Cont.

[d]Exclusive of the presenting emotional problem at 43rd St.

[e]Psychiatric prevalence is expected to be low in a child population over half of whose members were under six years of age.

Structure and Function of the Center

In addition to developing patient data, the HNP research staff conducted interviews with all members of the staff and attempted an overall appraisal of the function of the unit. Anyone applying for service is seen within a week, and more usually within 24 hours, after application. On evenings and weekends, however, the patient is seen at the centralized emergency service of the Consortium and then directed to the clinic the following morning.

The 43rd Street Center provides direct therapeutic services. These include crisis intervention, individual counseling, group therapy, psychiatric evaluation and referral, maintenance on medication, and referral to other social agencies. In addition, the center becomes a filter within the agency for referring patients to the inpatient and partial hospitalization services, and services for addictive diseases, for children, for the elderly, and for the retarded.

As part of its outreach program, the center works with local schools, police, and social agencies, as well as with medical providers. It shares clients with several agencies, particularly the Department of Public Welfare.

The HNP staff felt that as a self-contained unit, the center appears to function smoothly and cohesively without internal division. Morale is high, as is the sense of commitment. Unfavorable internal comments focus on the inadequacy of the current case notes and a need to specialize the intake function, which is currently rotated. The staff is also aware of a need for a higher level of training, better case assignment, and more vigorous follow up of cases. The need for specialized group therapy and community organization personnel is expressed.

The major perceived weak links, both as seen by HNP and Consortium personnel, appear when the ability of the system to work for the patient in a holistic fashion is tested. A significant problem within the Consortium is the lack of administrative connection between inpatient units and the centers. Current patterns also create a situation in which a first-year psychiatry resident can overrule the most senior psychiatric clinician in the Consortium in the matter of admitting a patient to the hospital. In addition, patients can get lost in the process of intraagency referral, and this type of problem is exaggerated in interagency dealings.

The HNP documents the tremendous difficulties encountered in the planning of holistic care [4,5,6]. An agency's perceptions of an applicant are

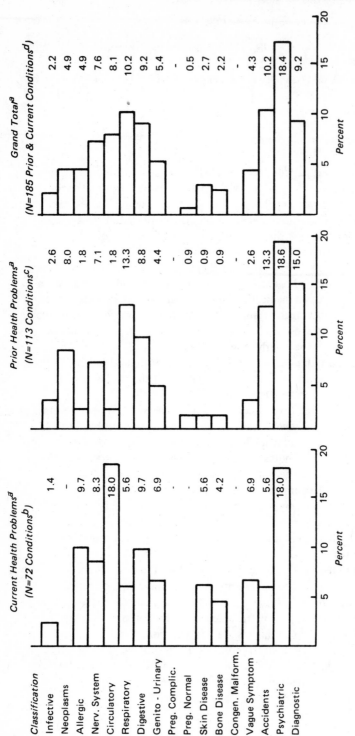

Classification	Current Health Problems[a] (N=72 Conditions[b])	Prior Health Problems[a] (N=113 Conditions[c])	Grand Total[a] (N=185 Prior & Current Conditions[d])
Infective	1.4	2.6	2.2
Neoplasms	-	8.0	4.9
Allergic	9.7	1.8	4.9
Nerv. System	8.3	7.1	7.6
Circulatory	18.0	1.8	8.1
Respiratory	5.6	13.3	10.2
Digestive	9.7	8.8	9.2
Genito - Urinary	6.9	4.4	5.4
Preg. Complic.	-	-	-
Preg. Normal	-	0.9	0.5
Skin Disease	5.6	0.9	2.7
Bone Disease	4.2	0.9	2.2
Congen. Malform.	-	-	-
Vague Symptom	6.9	2.6	4.3
Accidents	5.6	13.3	10.2
Psychiatric	18.0	18.6	18.4
Diagnostic	-	15.0	9.2

Source: Health Network Project Sample, 43rd Street Counseling Center, 1971.

[a]I.E., excludes emotional problem for which initial counseling center visit was made.

[b]Reported by 48 patients specifying one, two, or three conditions. Excludes presenting problem.

[c]One or more conditions reported by 71 patients. Includes two most recent problems for which treatment was received together with untreated problem within past year.

[d]One or more conditions reported by patients. Combines current health problems and prior conditions. Excludes presenting problem.

Figure 13-2. Current and prior health problems reported by 43rd Street Center patients by classification exclusive of

Table 13-5

Selected Interportal Data for Health Network Project Samples of Clients/Patients and Households

Other Problems, Staff Assessments, and External Referrals

	Portal				
Housing and Neighborhood Problems of Clients/Pts.	*Receiving Ward*	*CBA West*	*43rd Street*	*Child Welfare*	*All Portals*
Units in poor condition (major repairs)	18.9	18.9	14.5	18.0	17.9
Specific complaints re neighborhood	48.3	35.6	46.5	22.1[a]	38.7
Neighborhood not good for kids/aged	50.3	49.3	46.2	NA	–
Coping probs. of elderly and limited ambulatory problems	57.9	54.6	40.0	NA	–
Restriction in leaving house	51.3	51.5	40.0	NA	–
Sample children or children of sample adults with school adjustment problems	33.3	36.4	20.0	47.1	36.3
Clients/pts with legal probs.	NA	13.4	17.2	60.7[a]	–
Staff Assessments					
Need for further treatment or service for presenting problem	99.4	60.1[b]	90.4	89.0[a]	86.7
Presenting problem at moderate to acute severity at survey end	38.5	34.3	47.0	63.6[a]	46.2
Poor health an obstacle to economic self-sufficiency	65.5	39.4	78.9	58.0[a]	58.9
Clients/Patients referred outside portal system[c]	5.7	14.2	8.0	27.9[a]	13.5

Source: Health Network Project, Department of Community Medicine, University of Pennsylvania School of Medicine 1971.

Note: All figures are percents.

[a]The statistical unit is the child welfare family. The statistical unit in the other portals is the individual client or patient.

[b]Need for service *beyond* the basic need for financial support via the public assistance grant.

[c]Referrals include a small number of self initiated as opposed to agency initiated contacts. Referrals *exclude* contacts *within* portal systems, e.g., clinic referrals from Receiving Ward and Child Welfare purchase arrangements. In the case of Child Welfare the data refer to completed referrals.

Table 13-6
Duration of Current Health Problems Reported by 43rd Street
Patients Exclusive of Presenting Problem

	Conditions[a]	
Duration	Number	Percent
Under 1 month	9	17.6
1 to 6 months	10	19.6
6 months to 1 year	2	3.9
1 to 2 years	5	9.8
2 to 5 years	6	11.8
5 years or more	19	37.3
Total	51	100.0
Unknown	21	

Source: Health Network Project, Department of Community Medicine,
University of Pennsylvania School of Medicine—Sample, 43rd Street
Counseling Center, 1971.

[a]At least 37 patients reporting duration of one, two or three current
health problems.

Table 13-7
Duration of Prior Treated Health Problems Reported by 43rd
Street Patients

	Conditions[a]	
Duration	Number	Percent
Under 1 month	11	11.1
1 month to 6 months	15	15.2
6 months to 1 year	15	15.2
1 to 2 years	18	18.2
2 to 5 years	11	11.1
5 years or more	29	29.2
Total	99	100.0
Unknown	10	

Source: Health Network Project, Department of Community Medicine,
University of Pennsylvania School of Medicine—Sample, 43rd Street
Counseling Center, 1971.

[a]At least 68 patients reporting dureation of their two most recently
treated health problems. Current problems, treated or untreated, are
excluded.

colored by its own orientation, which may redefine his problems: the patient entering a medical portal finds his problems defined as medical, and so forth. This problem is compounded by the "territoriality" of agencies—their jealous guarding of their own turf. There is no guarantee that the patient's care will be maximized, and there are substantial and perhaps insurmountable barriers against establishing a central entry point or a common mechanism to best match patient/client needs with available services [3,4,7,8] .

In terms of the relationship between 43rd Street and Consortium head-quarters, two factors deserve note—communication and goal structure. The emphasis on decentralization is reflected in these factors: as the center is "distant" enough to pursue its own directions, it likewise is sufficiently "far" to have a sense of isolation from headquarters and, despite feeling it has some impact on headquarters' thinking, generally feels it learns of many decisions "after the fact," and perceives many directives as unclear. This remains the case despite headquarters staff's field visits and the center director's attending and reporting back on weekly headquarter's sessions. One might speculate that group and organizational forces act to frustrate rather than enhance communication efforts.

On another level, a marked discrepancy exists between the center and head-quarter's goal structures. When asked about future goals, administrative and supervisory center staff speak in terms of enhanced community outreach and expanded group services. Increased quality of care, via staff-departmental in-service training, is mentioned, and the means proposed are more personnel, more funds, and clearer enunciation of overall policy. Center personnel with treatment responsibility also articulate the need for "a comprehensive health care delivery system of which mental health services would be a part rather than the core."[4]

Upper echelon headquarters staff, however, focus on achieving quality treatment, facilitating the referral process, staff development, and the attempt to combine in one system care for emotional and physical problems. It is evident that those in headquarters are not spontaneously voicing interest or support for the center's high priority of expanding its specialized staff (which would enhance the center's autonomous strength), and that the center's administrator is not verbalizing the headquarters' priority of working toward an inclusive and comprehensive system (in which the center, per se, would perforce surrender its autonomy.) This is most dramatically reflected in the center's virtual lack of interaction with the Public Health unit in the same building. The direct treatment staff, without administrative and/or supervisory responsibilities, perhaps less concerned with the "turf" of the center, voices an interest in a comprehensive care system.

Discussion

It is, of course, not possible to generalize from one study. At best, one gets a snapshot of the function of one local neighborhood mental health clinic at one point in time. Nevertheless, discussions with directors of other such clinics in Philadelphia and elsewhere suggest that the data presented here are not unique. Certainly the 43rd Street Center fails in its mission to provide total comprehensive service to its clientele. Indeed, its registrants emerge as members of a population with an aggregation of problems and a cluster of needs which may far transcend the ability of a mental health entry point to meet them. Of this center's clients, 55 percent suffered from multiple conditions, that is, from problems beyond their presenting complaint; and 43 percent had medical problems, most of them chronic.

Despite ample availability of services in West Philadelphia, 18 percent of the sample indicated the persistence of conditions either untreated or without recent treatment. Health and mental health care was largely intermittent, and dental care largely absent. Although these patients entered a portal oriented along psychosocial dimensions offering psychotherapy as its service, the clients' needs go far beyond this portal's range of services. Despite this, the mental health system studied here referred only a very small percentage of its patients to outside care systems. and systematic follow up was lacking.

The HNP data reveal that for the 43rd Street Center and the other studied portals:

1. The full spectrum of client/patient needs for services are not being identified appropriately, much less being met.
2. For the population studied, problems tend to cluster in groups.
3. The primary purpose of the agency affects perceptions of the problems by the staff, shaping service delivery largely in line with agency purpose and bias rather than in conformity with the cluster of needs affecting the client/patient.
4. Linkages among agencies are ineffective in assisting in the processes of problem identification, solution, or case disposition.
5. Jurisdictional problems are of such magnitude that no comprehensive intake screening device alone will overcome them.

In summary, data from the HNP study of the 43rd Street Counseling Center of the West Philadelphia Community Mental Health Consortium indicate that even a well-functioning and well-accepted local neighborhood mental health center is a fragmentary provider to its consumers. Problems occur in cluster, and despite agency perceptions of their caseload as consumers of mental health care, consumer needs, when objectively researched, are not matched by the range of services the center provides or arranges. The center has not managed to interact with other components of the area's care providers to create a comprehensive system; general differences in organizational process as well as the value placed on decentralization by the center stand as barriers to this. In sum, agency perceptions, values, and need have more impact on service organization than the actual needs of the consumer population. A similar set of statements could be made about the other portals studied.

If the data from this single study can be replicated or confirmed in other ways, it will be necessary for deliverers of mental health services to acknowledge the failure of the local neighborhood mental health center as an effective overall delivery system for a population defined as "psychiatric." Indeed, as increasing attention is directed to the appreciation that social change is not synonymous with mental health care, and that community mental health centers as a group have wandered far outside their areas of competence, it is difficult to avoid questioning the continuing relevance of the free-standing community mental health center as an institution. With the full awareness of its current status as merely a partial provider of service, comes a sense of the need to link the center with a more comprehensive center, or to allow it and the contributions it has made to disappear.

To return to the questions posed earlier. Unfortunately, the data presented by the HNP shed no light on the matter of cost. However, a little arithmetic demonstrates that services in such a unit are delivered at relatively high cost. More important is the question of response to local needs. One can interpret the data at hand either positively or negatively. On balance, however, considerable and increasing response to these needs has occurred in the unit studied. All indications, however, show that the service is fragmentary. One must then ask the question, "Can the responsiveness of the neighborhood center be maintained if it is linked more appropriately with other services?" This might be accomplished in a number of ways. The community mental health center could conceivably expand into an all-purpose agency by including within itself medical services and relevant social components. But is mental health the proper auspice for such a generalized service? Alternatively, the CMHC could merge into the general welfare system and disappear as an entity.

Both of these alternatives seem harsh. A more viable option is being developed in northeastern Pennsylvania with the development of the United Service Agency (USA), in which all welfare, health, and mental health services are merging into one service unit. However, it took a major catastrophe in the area to induce agencies to give up their territories. A more immediately available choice is that of becoming a partner in the general health care system.

Conclusions

The nation's health care delivery system is in the process of major changes and realignments, and while its final form cannot yet be discerned, it is reasonably certain that vastly different patterns of providing both health care and financing of such care will be constructed. It is crucial that the community mental health center realistically assess its capabilities and strengths, as well as its weaknesses, and make contributions based on the painful lessons of its experience toward the evolution of a stronger health care delivery system. The strengths and weaknesses of the local mental health clinic described here may well prove to be an adequate testing ground for the model of a health care delivery system large enough to be comprehensive and small enough to be in touch with its community or consumer. If the lessons of the mental health field are heeded, the task of developing such a neighborhood unit will be a difficult one, since it must be seen as committed and concerned by the community, and yet not sacrifice the care of the whole human being.

Factors intrinsic to each type of unit suggest that the crucial issue is not necessarily the enforcement of centralization or decentralization but, rather, meaningful linkage and fruitful interdependence. It appears most judicious to accept the neighborhood center for what it is—a limited facility with many desirable attributes—and maximize its potential for productive interdigitation with closely related central units which are not solely mental-health oriented. In the long run, the neighborhood center, at high unit cost, may prove to accomplish things which a central unit would do for less, but is structurally and politically unable to do at all.

References

1. Department of Community Medicine Health Network Project, School of Medicine, University of Pennsylvania, *The Status of Community Mental Health Centers as an Element of Human Services.* Unpublished ms.

2. Leopold, R. L., Chapter in Bellak, Leopold, ed., *Progress in Community Mental Health*, 2nd ed., in preparation.

3. Leopold, R. L., "Urban Problems and the Community Mental Health Center: Multiple Mandates, Difficult Choices, 1. Background and Current Status," *American Journal of Orthopsychiatry*, 41, Jan., 1971, pp. 144-149.

4. Department of Community Medicine Health Network Project, School of Medicine, University of Pennsylvania, *The Agency Study-Health Network Project.* Unpublished ms.

5. Department of Community Medicine Health Network Project, School of Medicine, University of Pennsylvania, *The Client/Patient Survey-Health Network Project.* Unpublished ms.

6. Department of Community Medicine Health Network Project, School of Medicine, University of Pennsylvania, *The Health Network Project—Background, Methodology, Summary, Findings, Conclusions, and Recommendations.* Unpublished ms.

7. Brody, S. J., "The Law and the Health and Social Service Delivery Systems: A Study of Linkages." *Proceedings of Symposium on Law and the Aging, Syracuse University College of Law and the All-University Gerontology Center.* In press.

8. Leopold, E. A. and Schein, L., "Non-Accountability in the Human Services Non-System," *American Journal of Orthopsychiatry* 43, March, 1973.

14 Teaching and Learning Designs for Neighborhood Mental Health

Sandra Sutherland Fox

The provision of adequate and appropriate mental health services to people in their own communities and neighborhoods requires thoughtfully planned and often specialized training for the persons who work as staff or volunteers in a direct helping relationship to others. Knowledge, attitudes, and skills needed for effective and efficient delivery of neighborhood mental health services must be identified, taught, and learned in ways that not only render them theoretically understandable, but also allow for their broadest development as usable tools. Only in this way can competence combine with sense of commitment of persons working in the field of neighborhood mental health.

The Learners

Designers of training for providers of neighborhood mental health services must identify who is to be trained, what the training is to include, and how it is to be designed, conducted, and evaluated. Teaching-learning designs for staff and volunteers engaged in providing neighborhood mental health services must take into account the needs of workers for *specific* knowledge, attitudes, and skills. The challenge to the person responsible for training is to develop and bring into being learning experiences that address themselves to these areas of need.

The community caregivers in any neighborhood include the traditional mental health professionals as well as those who, without professional training in mental health, work as staff or volunteers in a direct helping relationship to others. Using this definition, neighborhood mental health workers include not only psychiatrists, psychologists, social workers, and psychiatric nurses, but also teachers, clergy, public welfare workers, probation officers, day care teachers, and aides, counselors, crisis intervention workers, and many others engaged in the helping process. Their learning needs range from seminars and workshops which will meet licensing and credentialing requirements to topical and skill-focused training for mental health professionals and nonprofessionals. Such training includes staff development and other continuing education programs which will update and upgrade knowledge and skills.

The responses to these and many related issues have resulted in a proliferation of training programs designed to have affective, behavioral, and/or cognitive learning outcomes. Lectures, t-groups, adult basic education courses, sensitivity training, and other models and methodologies have been used for training with little attention to who was being trained or what learning needs or competencies were being addressed. Many of these programs had good outcomes, and much was also learned from those that did *not* achieve the desired objectives. Accounts of these programs are available in the mental health and education literature [1-10]. Training programs were often designed quickly in order to respond to the requirements of funding grants; sometimes training was possible only after the mental health worker had been on his job in the neighborhood for weeks or months.

Adult Learning

Many training programs have not achieved their desired outcomes for neighborhood mental health workers because they failed to take into account the unique characteristics of adult learners. In order to be truly effective, learning experiences for adults must be different from the educational experiences most people have as children. The work of Malcolm Knowles has been useful in conceptualizing a theoretical base for adult learning, called "andragogy" [11]. Knowles describes four characteristics of the adult learner which have implications for the development of training programs for neighborhood mental health workers.

1. *Self-concept*: As a person matures, his self-concept changes from seeing himself as dependent to seeing himself as self-directing and autonomous. He wants to take responsibility for himself and resists learning under conditions which challenge his concept of himself as an independent person.
2. *Experience*: The adult learner has a reservoir of experience which he can draw on in his learning. Children must often learn by hearing about the experiences of adults, but the adult can relate his new learning to his own experience or to that shared by other adult learners.
3. *Readiness to Learn:* The adult's readiness to learn is related to the developmental tasks of his role. People learn best the things they need to know in order to advance from one phase of development to another. Each developmental task brings with it a "readiness to learn" that at its peak presents a "teachable moment."
4. *Time Perspective*: The time perspective of the adult focuses on immediate rather than postponed application of his learning. Also, the adult shifts his orientation from subject-centeredness to program-centeredness. Adults engage in learning in response to pressure they feel from current life problems; they want to apply their learning immediately.

Knowles has also developed a seven-step program planning process based on adult learning theory which can be used by trainers as a guide in designing teaching-

learning experiences for neighborhood mental health workers [12]. The steps
are as follows:

1. Establishment of a climate conducive to adult learning.
2. Creation of an organizational structure for mutual planning.
3. Diagnosis of learning needs.
4. Formulation of learning objectives.
5. Development of a design of learning activities.
6. Conduct of the learning experience.
7. Rediagnosis of learning needs.

Effective and efficient training for all levels and types of neighborhood mental
health workers will take into account characteristics of adult learners and the
andragogical process of program planning. In this way, training comes to have
genuine "felt" relevance to the experience of workers delivering mental health
services each day to neighborhood people.

The remainder of this chapter describes an attempt to put these principles
to work in a skill-focused training program for persons lacking professional
education in mental health and in a program of training for trainers, both of
which represent designs which can be used in teaching and learning for neighborhood mental health.

The Metropolitan Mental Health Skills Center [a]

The Metropolitan Mental Health Skills Center (MMHSC), a project of the Washington School of Psychiatry in Washington, D.C., provides continuing education for
persons who, without professional training in mental health, work as staff or
volunteers in a direct helping relationship to others. Participants in MMHSC
programs bring with them to training a wide range of educational backgrounds,
employment experiences, and life situations. Many work in a variety of
neighborhood-based settings. Their unifying characteristics are their wish to
develop skills for helping people and their lack of professional mental health
education. They may have had professional education in other fields such as
nursing, education, or law; they may be persons who have not yet completed
high school; or they may fall anywhere between these two points on the
educational continuum.

The choice as a target group for training of persons currently working as
staff or volunteers in a direct helping relationship to others and of persons without professional training in mental health is based on several factors. In the

[a]Partial support for the program of the Metropolitan Mental Health Skills Center was provided by Grant No. 21T15 MH11447, Public Health Service, National Institute of Mental
Health.

metropolitan Washington area, a number of "new careers" training programs are in operation which prepare people for entry-level jobs in mental health and the human services. A number of colleges and universities also offer professional training for social workers, psychiatrists, psychologists, and psychiatric nurses. Local chapters of professional associations for all of the mental health professions exist in the area. These educational institutions and professional groups represent a rich continuing education resource for the mental health professional. The remaining group of mental health workers — those other than new careerists or the traditional mental health professionals — comprise a large and varied group, already actively involved in providing services, whose training needs must be met if neighborhood mental health services are to be adequate and appropriate. It is to this group that the Metropolitan Mental Health Skills Center has given priority. Students include persons working in such jobs as counselors, corrections officers, day care staff, public health and visiting nurses, clergy, teachers, neighborhood workers, case aides, public welfare workers with a bachelor's degree or less, lawyers in neighborhood agencies, friendly visitors, volunteers in local mental association programs, and residential child care staff. When spaces are available, registration for MMHSC seminars and workshops is opened to mental health professionals who, interestingly, say they never had skill-focused courses in their graduate education. The Center currently offers one seminar, entitled Supervision of the Nonprofessional, which is available on an open registration basis both to persons without professional training in mental health and to mental health professionals.

A distinguishing feature of the Metropolitan Mental Health Skills Center is its emphasis on skill training. Initial ideas and impressions about the appropriateness of this focus have been confirmed by experience. Students come to MMHSC programs asking "What do I do?" or "What do I say?" in particular situations in which they are the helping person. The Center's initial focus on specific skills, followed by attention to the theory that underpins the skill and the ways in which the skill can be generalized to other situations is what Center students say has made these learning experiences meaningful for them and has motivated them to return for additional training. They see the Center as interested in helping them to provide good service to the people they work with every day, to understand the theory that explains the dynamics of a situation, and to translate their newly acquired skills from a particular situation or problem to more general usefulness. In focusing on skills first and theory later, training offered at MMHSC is the reverse of the way many persons learned in the past. Usually initial attention is given to theory, and if time permits (which it often does not), consideration is given to the application of the theories in actual situations.

The Metropolitan Mental Health Skills Center offers fifteen to twenty seminars and three to six workshops in each of its catalogues, published two or three times a year and mailed to approximately 7,500 individuals and agencies in metropolitan Washington. Seminars, limited to 15 participants, meet for about two hours per week for eight to twelve weeks. These seminars consider such topics as: Diagnostic Thinking and Planning, Use of Self in the Helping Process, Working with Groups, Designing Activity Programs to Respond to Emotional Needs, and Helping People Cope with Separation and Loss.

The Diagnostic Thinking and Planning seminar, for example, works toward the following learning objectives: differentiating facts from interpretations, defining the client's basic problem (as differentiated from the symptoms of the problem), determining realistic goals, developing a working agreement with the client, and designing a plan to meet the agreed upon goals. Seminar participants write process records of their own difficult interviews, study written and tape recorded interviews, participate in short, skill-focused exercises, read popular paperback books about people and problems (such as *Captain Newman, M.D., One Flew Over the Cuckoo's Nest, Up the Down Staircase, Pimp: The Story of My Life,* and *Can't You Hear Me Talking to You* [13-17] present a reaction to what they have read, determine appropriate referral resources for a person with a specific problem, and participate in group discussions.

Workshops, generally limited to 35 to 40 persons, meet for one or two full days. They consider such topics as Death and the Dying Client, Fostering Creativity in Children, Evaluating Mental Health Needs of the Elderly, and Building the Self Concept. The six-hour workshop, Evaluating Mental Health Needs of the Elderly, for example, includes a brief didactic presentation by the workshop leader, discussion of the presentation, a live interview of an elderly person by the workshop leader to illustrate interviewing and content issues, and small discussion groups to consider application of what has been learned to the participant's own work situation.

Seminars attract persons interested in and with time for more extensive and intensive skill development. The shorter workshops have more limited objectives and permit people to test out their interest in returning to a learning situation, perhaps after years away from or after educational experiences which have left a residue of negative feelings.

In order to encourage enrollment, the tuition for seminars and workshops is kept at a level comparable to fees for public adult education, and scholarships are available for persons whose financial situation would otherwise make participation impossible. MMHSC seminars and workshops have been subsidized in part by a grant from the National Institute of Mental Health Continuing Education Branch and also by grants from private foundations and interested individuals.

In addition to its publicly offered seminars and workshops, the Center designs and conducts inservice training and staff development programs for various agencies or groups. This training is developed to meet the specific skill content and time requirements of the requesting group, which is expected to meet the actual cost of the training to the maximum extent possible.

The Metropolitan Mental Health Skills Center also offers an eight-course

Certificate Program designed to develop in the participant a core of basic mental health skills applicable to a wide range of typical mental health problems and a variety of age groups. Three seminars (or approved equivalents) are required in the Certificate Program: Diagnostic Thinking and Planning, Use of Self in the Helping Process, and The Tasks of Development. Of the additional five courses, one must relate to work with children, one to work with adolescents or young adults, and one to work with adults; the other two courses are electives, to be selected by the Certificate Program student according to his or her own particular interests. Four workshops may be used as an alternate to one seminar to meet the requirement of one of these latter five courses. The Certificate Program also requires participation in a "Consultation Semester" during which the student must design, conduct, and discuss a project which he and the Center staff agree will demonstrate his ability to integrate, label, and use the knowledge, attitudes, and skills he has learned in his MMHSC courses.

The MMHSC administrative staff is small — two professionals (who also teach seminars for the Center) and a secretary, who is also the registrar for seminars and workshops. Each semester the faculty includes approximately fifteen experienced mental health practitioners selected because of their ability to conceptualize and teach mental health skills and because of their belief in the important contributions which can be made by mental health workers who lack formal professional mental health training. Most faculty lead an MMHSC seminar or workshop in addition to their regular employment. The Center holds monthly faculty meetings which provide an opportunity for sharing information and ideas about the Center. In addition, these meetings are used for discussion of specific teaching and learning issues as they arise in various seminars, workshops, and inservice training programs. These discussions have included such concerns as: how to teach skills, dealing with hostile or disruptive students, translating clinical experience into teachable units, developing measurable objectives for a particular course, and handling unexpected student reaction to a faculty member's planned absence from one of the middle sessions of a seminar. Faculty receive an honorarium for their teaching. Most say they have found their MMHSC experience very challenging and exciting, and they look forward to teaching in succeeding semesters and to working with students who seem so eager to learn.

The Center for Creative Teaching

The Center for Creative Teaching (CCT), focusing on adult teaching and learning in mental health and the human services, is also a project of the Washington School of Psychiatry in Washington, D.C. After it had been established approximately seven years, MMHSC staff realized the Skills Center was training approximately 1,000 students a year and had a waiting list of approximately 1,000 students seeking training. A review of these trainees and applicants revealed that many came from agencies with existing training or staff development personnel or departments. People from these agencies reported that training programs offered at their agencies were poorly designed and conducted, however, and that staff were often forced to attend training sessions selected for them by supervisors and administrators rather than sessions staff felt would help them in their work. Therefore, whenever possible, staff from these agencies came to MMHSC rather than attending programs offered by their own agencies.

In an attempt to reduce its waiting list and to strengthen existing mental health and human services training programs in the community, MMHSC established a "Training for Trainers" program. It is this program which has recently been incorporated into the new Center for Creative Teaching, formally established in December, 1975 as a program with a broader base than that of the Skills Center.

The Center for Creative Teaching is dedicated to the concept that good training programs require well trained educators and trainers in order to have an impact on the delivery of neighborhood mental health services. As good teaching and learning situations are made available to mental health workers, one can expect to see a direct impact on the diagnostic, therapeutic, and preventive services they provide. Good learning and teaching bears a direct relationship to good trainers.

The goals of the Center for Creative Teaching are: (1) To develop a cadre of persons able to design, conduct, and evaluate sound education and training programs in the fields of mental health and the human services; (2) To design and share on a local, regional, and national level a replicable model for the training of persons with responsibility for teaching those working in the mental health and human service fields; (3) To provide continuing education programs and activities to extend and enhance the knowledge, attitudes, and skills of mental health and human services teachers and trainers; and (4) To publish materials for use in the training and ongoing work of mental health and human services teachers and trainers.

Programs and services offered and projected by CCT include a Two-Year Certificate Program for Educators and Trainers, Seminars and Workshops, Agency-Based Training for Trainers Programs, a Monthly Forum for Mental Health and Human Service Educators, Local, Regional, and National Conferences, and Publications.

The Certificate Program, for example, requiring six hours each semester for four semesters, includes a didactic seminar, (the Self As Educator seminar) and either observations or a practicum each semester. The program design for the two years is as follows:

1st Year

Program Planning for Adult Learners (1st semester): program planning skills for adult learning; delineation of the program planning process; design of a training program to be conducted during the second semester.

Teaching Methodology and Materials for Adult Learners (2nd semester): various materials and approaches and the values and limitations of each.

Self As Educator – I & II (1st and 2nd semesters): exploration of the role of teacher or trainer and its comforts and discomforts; the use of self in the teaching-learning transaction.

Observation (1st semester): planned observation of an adult learning program.

Practicum I (2nd semester): conduct training program designed during first semester.

2nd year

Evaluation of Mental Health and Human Services Continuing Education Programs (1st semester, half semester): designing and conducting appropriate evaluation of programs.

Skill Elective (1st semester, half semester): to be chosen from CCT offerings.

Administering Continuing Education Programs (2nd semester): selection of students, faculty development, target groups, financing, relationships with community and agencies.

Self As Educator – III & IV (1st and 2nd semesters): continuation from first year.

Practicum II (1st and 2nd semesters). design, conduct, and evaluate a longer, more complex teaching-learning experience. Written report on Practicum II is required for graduation and certification.

Participants in the Certificate Program include a day care center director with staff training responsibilities, a volunteer corps director from a local mental health association, a psychiatric nurse who is responsible for training LPNs on their rotation through the psychiatric unit of a local hospital, and a doctoral student with an LEAA grant to develop a training design and materials for child care workers in group homes for adjudicated adolescent girls.

Seminars and workshops offered on an individual registration basis by CCT include all Certificate Program didactic seminars (extra spaces are opened for registration by persons not enrolled in the Certificate Program) as well as; Teaching by Interviewing; Things Learners Remember: Locating, Selecting, and Effectively Using Illustrative and Thought-Provoking Teaching Materials; and Teaching-Learning Issues and Problems in Hotline and Telephone Crisis Intervention Training Programs.

The Center for Creative Teaching represents an effort to make a direct impact on the delivery of neighborhood mental health services by training trainers rather than continually expanding direct training opportunities for caregivers. This approach strengthens training offered by local agencies and programs and permits resources such as the Metropolitan Mental Health Skills Center to provide educational experiences for staff and volunteers who otherwise have no such training available and to offer specialized training programs which cannot be conducted by the local agencies.

Summary

The neighborhood mental health movement has many implications for the design of teaching and learning programs. We have learned to listen to the needs and hopes of clients and patients; designers and deliverers of training programs must now learn to listen to the self-diagnosed learning needs of the wide range of staff and volunteers providing neighborhood mental health services.

The programs of the Metropolitan Mental Health Skills Center and the Center for Creative Teaching have been presented as possible models for training programs responsive to the learning needs of neighborhood mental health workers. The programs are effective and appropriate because they take into account in their design and conduct the unique characteristics of adult learners and because they follow a program planning process which involves the adult learner and asks him to take responsibility for his own learning. These programs involve teaching and learning designs for specific kinds and levels of neighborhood mental health workers and are directly related to the roles and tasks of those workers. Each program is intended to have a direct impact on the delivery of neighborhood mental health services through improved quality care as a result of increased and refined skills among mental health workers and through an expansion of the pool of individuals trained to provide local services. Neighborhood mental health programs will need to organize similar training efforts themselves or relate to free-standing programs such as those described here.

References

1. Barr, S. "Some Observations on the Practice of Indigenous Nonprofessional Workers," Paper presented at the Council on Social Work Education Annual Program Meeting, January, 1966.

2. Christmas, J. J. "Group Methods in Training and Practice: Nonprofessional Mental Health Personnel in a Deprived Community," *American Journal of Orthopsychiatry*, *36*, 410-19. April, 1966.

3. Godenne, G.D. "Mental Hygiene Seminars for School Personnel: Report of a Pilot Project". *Public Health Reports*, *81*, 348-50, April 1966.

4. Hines, L. "A Nonprofessional Discusses Her Role in Mental Health," *American Journal of Psychiatry*, *126*, 1467-72, April, 1970.

5. Johnson, D. and Ferryman, Z.C. "Inservice Training for Nonprofessional Personnel in a Mental Retardation Center," *Mental Retardation*, 7, 10-13, October, 1969.

6. Kadish, J. "Mental Health Training of Police Officers," *Mental Hygiene*, 50, 205-10, April, 1966.

7. Levenson, A.I., Beck, J.C., Quinn, R., Putnam. P. "Manpower and Training in Community Mental Health Centers," *Hospital and Community Psychiatry*, 20, 85-88, March 1969.

8. Mandeville, P.F. and Maholick, L.T. "Changing Points of Emphasis in Training the Community's Natural Counselors," *Mental Hygiene, 53,* 208-13, 1969.

9. Hoch, M., Elkes, D., Flint, A.A. *Pilot Project in Training of Mental Health Counselors.* Washington, D.C.: U.S. Department of Health, Education and Welfare. Public Health Service Publication No. 1254, undated.

10. Shapiro, D.S., Maholick, L.T., and Robertson, R.N. "Mental Health Training for Ministers," *American Journal of Public Health*, 57, 518-22, March, 1967.

11. Knowles, M. S. *The Modern Practice of Adult Education: Andragogy versus Pedagogy.* New York: Association Press, 1970, pp. 39-49.

12. Knowles, M. S. "Program Planning for Adults as Learners," *Adult Leadership,* February, 1967.

13. Rosten, L. *Captain Newman, M.D.* Greenwich, Connecticut: Fawcett (Crest Paperback R604), 1963.

14. Kesey, K. *One Flew Over the Cuckoo's Nest.* New York: The New American Library, (Signet Paperback Q4171), 1962.

15. Kaufman, B. *Up the Down Staircase.* New York: The Hearst Corporation. (Avon Paperback N130), 1964.

16. Slim, I. *Pimp: The Story of My Life.* Los Angeles: Holloway House Publishing Co. (Holloway House Paperback HH-139), 1969.

17. Mirthes, C., et al. *Can't You Hear Me Talking To You?* New York: Bantam Books (Bantam Books Paperback N5934), 1971.

15

Psychiatric Training in Neighborhood Settings

Steven S. Sharfstein
and *James E. Sabin*

As mental health services extend and decentralize into neighborhoods, training for neighborhood psychiatry poses special problems for the already heavily burdened psychiatric resident and the staff supervisor. The range of the "catchment area" patients, especially alcoholics, drug abusers, and elderly with chronic brain syndromes, place new demands on residents and staff supervisors for which training in traditional psychotherapy has few answers. Asking residents to leave the hospital and work in agencies whose priorities are not solely (and often not primarily) mental health is an additional stress that can confuse and discourage the young psychiatrist, who is unsure of his professional identity and the value of his work. At the same time, if we value the future of neighborhood psychiatry, it is essential to expose residents to this work early in training before role concepts are frozen and have become difficult to modify [1,2,3].

A description of one experiment in education follows. This program attempted to (1) attract psychiatric residents to neighborhood psychiatry, and (2) determine the real cost of this effort by evaluating the trade-off of training with service.

Description of the Program

In 1970, first year residents from one of four inpatient services of the Massachusetts Mental Health Center, a university affiliated community mental health and and retardation center, in Boston began to work directly in the community by spending four hours each week in a comprehensive neighborhood health center. In 1971, residents from the second inpatient service began to work at another neighborhood center, and in 1973 a third service was linked with a third center. This work became a required part of the residency curriculum.

At the centers, the residents worked with multiproblem families and provided crisis intervention and short-term psychotherapy. They participated in, and we hope learned about, how mental health services are designed for neighborhoods where there are practically no physicians and where the front-line mental health personnel are welfare workers, legal-aid lawyers, priests, schoolteachers, and employment counselors.

The residents had as their supervisor the director of mental health for the neighborhood center. A second-year resident served as coordinator, or chief resi-

Views expressed herein are those of the authors and do not necessarily reflect the opinions, official policies, or positions of the NIMH, ADAMHA, or the Harvard Community Health Plan.

dent, for the project. A program of case conferences with prestigious community psychiatrists was developed to supplement the conferences already well established as part of the teaching program for first-year residents.

In the first year of the program, residents came primarily as observers, since services were in the process of development. They observed mental health consultation and participated in crisis intervention. The second year shifted the focus to direct patient care by assigning multiproblem families to the residents for extended diagnostic and therapeutic planning. Responsibility for the family rested with the resident, and supervision closely resembled psychotherapy supervision in the hospital. We hoped that taking responsibility for a difficult case would create the right mix of anxiety and interest in order to maximize learning. Residents were expected to collaborate with health center paraprofessionals in the evaluation and treatment of the multiproblem family. In subsequent years of training, the residents, depending on their particular interests, had opportunities for both consultation and clinical work.

Examples of the activities of several residents follows. One resident was assigned a multiproblem, six-member family for evaluation and treatment, with the index case a depressed, pregnant 14 year old. Together with the psychiatric nurse and a paraprofessional worker, a treatment plan was worked out. Collaboration with the welfare worker became essential. In addition to working with an interdisciplinary and interagency team, the resident made home visits, provided family and crisis therapies, and struggled with a situation in almost constant turmoil. This resident also developed a basketball clinic one evening a week at a teen drop-in center and consulted with the parish priest who directed the center.

Another resident, in addition to working with a family in crisis due to the father's sudden unemployment, consulted in a nursing home — seeing cases with a social worker and meeting with the director and her staff. A third resident introduced himself to the community relations officer at the local police station and consulted with several policemen. A fourth resident, after an extended family evaluation, began treatment of an 8 year old child.

From July, 1970 to 1973, during each year, one second-year resident, as an elective, spent one-half to two-thirds time in one of the health centers seeing patients, consulting with center staff, and with one outside agency, acting as chief resident, and helping coordinate the teaching program for first-year residents.

The program offered a varied experience to residents on both a required and elective basis, with different forms of teaching and supervision. In an effort to evaluate the teaching program, a survey of supervisors and of 50 residents divided into two groups was administered in April of 1972 [4]. Of 25 first-year residents randomly selected to have experience in neighborhood settings, 40 percent continued this work into the second and third year of residency. Of 25 first-year residents with no such experience, only 8 percent subsequently worked or planned to work in any community setting. The supervisors were enthusiastic about teaching in the neighborhood where resident and supervisor could learn together as colleagues. Working together in the real field, with practical and theoretical issues constantly intermingled, residents and supervisors found a sense of immediacy and excitement in the educational process.

In sum then, although the first-year residents felt burdened by the time commitment at the neighborhood centers, they were pleased with their experience. However, the survey revealed the widely shared complaint that they found it difficult to understand the role of psychiatrists at the centers or the workings of the mental health program itself. Their own roles had been defined more by educational considerations than by the service needs of the center.

Instead of being assigned to a part of the center and exposed to whatever service demands came their way, the residents had been given selected clinical tasks, chosen for educational value. Most of the cases referred to them were multiproblem, disorganized individuals and families, who are often not selected at outpatient clinics that emphasize psychotherapeutic treatment. Such cases provided a challenging clinical experience. However, because of the very limited time spent at the centers, residents were not able to develop a network of relationships conducive to formal and informal consultation. As relative outsiders, they could not participate effectively in administration or program planning. This appears to have limited their understanding of the work the centers actually did and the psychiatrist's role in the overall program.

Cost-Accounting: Training vs. Service

One way to evaluate mental health services and teaching is a cost-accounting study [5]. In November of 1972 all staff and residents at one neighborhood health center were interviewed and asked to account for all time spent during a representative week. Teaching responsibilities were separated from learning time, but the combination accounted for the high cost of teaching. The cost-accounting study at the one neighborhood center revealed that teaching six part-time, first-year residents cost three times more per hour of service than using the same hour for staff personnel to provide direct service. A supervisory hour with a resident not only takes into account the supervisor's time but also the time of the resident or group of residents. A weekly workshop cost almost $100 an hour in staff and resident time. In evaluating whether this is "too much," we must ask ourselves if the benefit of this effort outweighs its high cost. Considering the data presented previously — that 40 percent of those with neighborhood exposure continue their community work and only 8 percent with no exposure enter this field — is this one-out-of-three "success ratio" (assuming some long-term validity) worth the price paid in loss of service time for senior staff? Who should decide on the acceptability of the trade-off of training and service, the residency-training program or the neighborhood board?

The issue is different in the training of community mental health workers. Here, neighborhood residents, often low-income people, embark on an upwardly mobile career ladder that is not only of benefit to the neighborhood in terms of service but also in terms of jobs and income. Thus the trade-offs for training local mental health workers are different from those associated with resident training.

In a setting as diffuse and egalitarian as the neighborhood health center, the first-year resident needs structure, close supervision, and therefore costly teaching. The cost of community teaching is high and perhaps unacceptable, given the priorities of the neighborhood. The second- and third-year resident, however, is in a much better position not only to understand and integrate the clinical and consultative experience but also to provide service that at least equals if not outweighs in value the cost of teaching. The advanced resident has a more solid grounding in diagnosis and treatment, as well as an identity as a therapist.

The need for psychiatrists to work in community and neighborhood settings is clear. Alternatives to private practice and institutional psychiatry must be presented early to young residents. Making this an attractive, understandable alternative is a major goal of teaching neighborhood psychiatry.

References

1. Morrison, A.P., Shore, M.F., and Grobman, J., "On the Stresses of Community Psychiatry and Helping Residents to Survive Them," *American Journal of Psychiatry 130,* 1237-1241, 1973.

2. Cotton, P.G. and Pruett, K.D., "The Affective Experience of Residency Training in Community Psychiatry," *American Journal of Psychiatry 132,* 267-270, 1975.

3. Sharfstein, S.S., Scherl, D.J., and Gault, W.B., "Incorporating Community Psychiatry in First-Year Residency Training," *Hospital and Community Psychiatry*, Vol. 23, February, 1972, pp. 38-40.

4. Sabin, J.E. and Sharfstein, S.S., "Integrating Community Psychiatry into Residency Training," *Hospital and Community Psychiatry,* Vol. 26, No. 5, May, 1975, pp. 289-292.

5. Sharfstein, S.S., "A Cost-Effectiveness Approach to Mental Health Service and Training in a Neighborhood Health Center." Unpublished study.

16

An Experimental Project in Training Neighborhood Mental Health Practitioners in the Resolution of Intergroup Conflict

Roberto L. Jimenez

Understanding and managing conflict between groups — whether between adolescent gangs, social classes, ethnic groups, races, or service staff and administration of a health center — is perhaps the most difficult challenge that neighborhood mental health practitioners encounter in their work. Such conflict is often deeply rooted in a complex interplay of personal, sociocultural, economic, religious, and historical forces that are as yet poorly understood. The practitioner, in searching for ways of mediating intergroup rivalries, must address himself to those factors in daily life that inhibit people from relating to one another and hence foster difficulties in communication. In addition, the practitioner must simultaneously seek means of resolving personal conflicts, many of which are on the hazy periphery of awareness or are totally unconscious. This dual task in conflict resolution calls for clinicians with sound backgrounds in both individual dynamics and the principles of social psychology and group behavior. It requires that the clinician understand the effects of contemporary society on psychological functioning, as well as how deeply rooted emotional problems blind one to certain aspects of human relationships.

The training of neighborhood mental health practitioners with psychosocial perspectives is a formidable task. Intergroup conflict and harmony is not a subject which lends itself readily to systematic study. The issues involved in such disputes are often too complex and varied for any one person to understand or manage fully. The mistrust, fear, and hostility often seem too volatile and unresponsive to any known psychotherapeutic intervention. The calm, sensitive but stern leadership that such conflict demands is a rare quality and extremely difficult to acquire.

In recent years, a new training methodology has been introduced which is said to hold the promise of studying intergroup conflict in ways that were never before possible. This measure, a form of experience-based learning, can be labeled with the generic term of "experiential groups." An "experiential group" is generally a small gathering of people in which interpersonal confrontations are fostered for the purpose of influencing and developing skills toward more productive social activity. The process is a mixture of social psychology, educational psychology, managerial techniques, and group psychotherapy. The experiential group cuts across many disciplines and brings them to bear on a small lifelike experience under controlled conditions. It thus offers a unique opportunity for developing the skills required for an effective neighborhood mental health care practice.

191

This chapter describes an experiment which attempted to elucidate and resolve an ongoing conflict between the professional social service staff and a
group of Hispanic neighborhood workers in a neighbrohood health center in the
Boston area. It was a one-year training experience in which a variety of human
service professionals and neighborhood workers participated from both inside and
outside the center in question. Most members of the group were fluent in Spanish
and English and over half were native Spanish-speaking. The participants were invited to undergo the experience at the request of the author who served as the
group leader. The project was offered as an accredited course at Boston University
and met weekly for two-and-one-half hour sessions.

History of the Group

The author was contacted by the director of social services in a neighborhood
health center where he was a consultant who sought his assistance in dealing with
several problems she was having concerning her Spanish-speaking community
workers. Her concern was that these workers were not being totally honest in discussing their cases with their supervisors. Often they would not notify their immediate supervisor about their wish to consult with the psychiatric consultant (this
author) about cases. Further, they would frequently supplant or alter suggestions that were made in regard to case management, without mentioning their
intentions to do so. They would also take it upon themselves to intervene in
ways which they deemed appropriate without discussion.

It was clear from the conversation that the director was involved in one of
the knottiest issues that develops between native Spanish-speaking mental health
care providers and those providers and supervisors who are not familiar with the
culture and issues of health care delivery in the Spanish-speaking community. To
assist the director, the author brought together the Spanish-speaking workers
involved. At the meeting, the Hispanic group expressed the opinion that the problem which existed between them and their supervisors was an unsolvable one. It
was their feeling that the professional staff of the department had never been
sincere in regard to providing services for the Spanish-speaking. As evidence, they
cited the fact that little effort had been made to acquaint themselves with the culture, language, or family life styles of the Spanish-speaking, and pointed to the
lack of Spanish-speaking professional staff and administrators as further proof of
their beliefs. They felt that the non-Spanish-speaking professional was incapable
of delivering adequate services to the Spanish-speaking, and had thus begun the
practice of utilizing their own "know-how" without discussion. It was their
contention that new, culturally appropriate methods of understanding and intervening were in order. Professional casework practices were deemed appropriate
only for the non-Spanish-speaking. They were adamant about not making available to "outsiders" whatever skills and knowledge they possessed or were de-

veloping. It was their feeling that the "professional staff" was more interested in "conducting conferences" and "writing papers" than in quality service.

The Hispanic staff was clearly frustrated, very angry, and felt exploited and powerless. Toward the latter part of the meeting, issues of conflicted identity and desires for upward mobility began to surface. The workers began to share with each other their personal struggles, hopes, problems, and ambitions. At this point the author suggested a city wide, on going forum where groups could gather and work on issues arising in neighborhood human service practice in the Spanish-speaking community. It was proposed that the experiment take place on "neutral ground" and that some form of "meaningful credit" be given to the participants. The workers responded enthusiastically, and urged proceeding as quickly as possible with the project. After a series of meetings it was decided that the author should lead and structure the experience as he saw fit.

Characteristics of the Group

The group consisted of twenty members and the author. Five of the members were bilingual professionals. Five other members were professionals who did not speak Spanish and had had relatively little exposure to human service issues in this Spanish-speaking community. Two native, Spanish-speaking human service professionals participated. Four Hispanic community workers from the health center under discussion were involved, as well as four other Hispanic neighborhood workers from other centers. The basic format was that of a task-oriented training group, designed to explore systematically the issues involved in practicing mental health skills in the Spanish-speaking community.

The mixture of members described above was deliberately chosen to create an atmosphere that would maximize the conflicts and dynamics which Spanish-speaking community workers had to face in their daily work. It was also decided that guests from a wide range of fields would be invited to participate in the group for certain periods of time. The group members were required to gather materials from their human service activities, from their reading and life experiences, and bring them to the group for discussion. The leader would set the agenda for the group and guide it toward fulfilling its goal. On occasions, there would be didactic teaching activities by the group leader, by the special guest, or by other people who would be designated to perform this task. The leader would visit each member at his or her work site on an ongoing basis throughout the week to assist in the process of gathering materials appropriate for the group and making observations of the application of the knowledge being generated by the group to their cases. It was decided that the experience would last about one year, that the group would meet once weekly for two-and-one-half hours, and that college credits at Boston University would be offered to those who wished to apply the experience towards a bachelor's or a master's program.

Group Process

The initial sessions were characterized by a burst of activities and enthusiasm.
Members were quick with ideas and topics for discussion. Lists were brought in
itemizing areas of concern. Such things as culture conflicts, social class conflicts,
upward mobility, identity assimilations, and migration were foremost on people's
minds. The Spanish-speaking workers were particularly concerned about discussing the consequences of cultural exclusion and its implications for character
formation and psychological illness. They also wanted very much to explore
Hispanic concepts of health and illness found in the rural and semirural areas
and their implications for treatment. There was considerable emphasis, by all
members, on exploring the Spanish-speaking family and its dynamics. The professionals were particularly concerned with the issues between supervisors and
supervisees and between professionals and nonprofessionals of different cultures.

Awareness and Division

As the group proceeded to analyze the wealth of initial materials and suggestions
so that the task for the remainder of the year could be constructed, the participants began to divide themselves into subgroups of similar interest and background — Hispanic professionals, bilingual professionals, non-Spanish-speaking
professionals; and native Spanish-speaking community workers. The participants
without prior human service experiences in the Spanish-speaking community
tended to isolate themselves and speak little. This division into subgroups happened without notice. Everyone was so eager and busy with the task at hand
that little attention was paid to the process.

As the agenda for the work that was to be accomplished was decided, the
group began to change its character. The Spanish-speaking community workers
began to take the initiative with comments aimed more at embarrassing the
non-Hispanic professionals than discussing the issues at hand. They would dwell
on minor points and use cultural explanations inappropriately. When an impasse
was reached over a solution to a particular problem, the community workers
would turn to the few Hispanic professionals present as if to seek a final word on
the subject, and these Hispanic professionals would usually respond with vague
and rather noncommittal answers. During the mid-session break and after each
session, the leader would be surrounded by the Hispanic community workers on
one side asking questions in Spanish and the non-Hispanic professionals on the
other side asking questions in English. The rest of the participants would stand
in the back of these two parties listening and anxiously awaiting some encourag-
ment from the leader that would allow them to get into the action.

Submergence

In time, all members began to isolate themselves from each other. One would note long periods of silence in the group, with frequent private conversations among the various members of the subgroups. Other significant events were absences by various group members. When the leader pointed out the phenomena of subdividing and absences, the group as a whole resisted dealing with the subject. For example, when the community workers were asked about the whereabouts of some of their peers, they generally would respond by saying that they had no idea why the absent members were not present. When the leader visited the various centers where the members worked he was greeted with a certain amount of indifference and coldness. Indirect messages, that is, messages by third parties, began to arrive. The leader was frequently approached by friends of the community workers and comments were made about the group. In general, the remarks centered around the dissatisfactions that the Spanish-speaking community workers were having with the group experience. It was their opinion that the leader was catering to the wishes and agendas of the professionals and not proving useful. Most of the community workers saw no point in the experience and felt that the discussions were too academic and lacked the realism they felt was necessary. They were experiencing doubt about continuing in the group. They were also quite annoyed at having to read a great deal of material in preparation for the group which they felt was useless for their clinical practice, and sensed an effort to make them uncomfortable when they presented their cases. They felt that they did not have to go to great length to explain their cases or to analyze them, and resented being asked to justify their interventions to people whom they felt had no particular interest in providing services to their clients. Their remarks also suggested anger at the group leader and a feeling of being let down. Most were unanimous in the opinion that it would be much more profitable to have a group composed exclusively of Spanish-speaking workers.

After much soul-searching, the leader drafted a letter to all the group members containing his analysis of the dynamics which included the following observations: that the group had reached a point in which the various members were becoming emotionally involved with one another and the members were beginning to wonder whether they really wanted to go through an experience that would demand sharing and taking risks. The leader reminded them about the purpose of the group. He told them that it had been designed to deal with the kinds of conflicts that were generated between providers and supervisors from different cultures. He reminded them that the group's purpose was to retrace, as much as possible, the conditions in which culture conflict evolves, and to explore them at both an intellectual and an emotional level. He pointed out how mutually adaptive responses are created, and challenged all members not to stop at this point. The letter ended by saying that it was vital to continue — to not lose the opportunity to explore whether providers from different cultures *could* in fact work together, or even begin to understand each other. The leader then made a point to visit as many individual group members as he could to discuss personally his letter with them and urge them to continue in the group. He also strongly urged that each make a commitment to the group for the next meeting.

This meeting was attended by all the members, and the leader discussed the letter which he had sent to them and elaborated on his interpretation of the events that had taken place up to that point. He then told the group that it was his wish that they be divided into subgroups of a mixed nature, with balance being the key element in this new arrangement. Each subgroup then would be given a specific assignment based on the materials that had been produced in the initial sessions. The subgroups were also told that each had to elect a leader of their own choosing whose task was to coordinate and direct the activities of the subgroup, paying attention to the guidelines and examples that had been set forth in the initial phases of the group. The plans were to reassemble these groups at a future point to compare findings and to share experiences. The leader's job was to circulate among these various subgroups, observe them, and assist them to accomplish their work.

Emergence

This intervention produced another spurt of intense and enthusiastic activity. When the group reconvened, the atmosphere was one of competition among the subgroups. Loyalty was clearly to other subgroup members and their leaders. Each, in turn, sought to obtain special attention from the leader during the session break. After each class, the members would surround him with questions that were directed through their subgroup leaders. The members of these subgroups would loosely align themselves behind their leaders in bringing in materials and urging their leader to seek attention. In time, subgrouping phenomena began to wane and members seemed to be more on their own. They began to seek the leader out individually, requesting advice on specific cases and human service practices, or clarification on some reading material that had been given to them at the beginning. Usually their requests or questions were filled with a good bit of personal data and an implicit wish that the leader respond with psychological insight and directions. The group, however, began to display much more interaction and sharing among members. Certain key people began to evolve as spokespersons, and members began to speak openly and frankly. Community workers and professionals seemed to accept each other more as equals, and discussions were more aggressive, but open.

It was at this point that the leader reminded the group of the impending termination and the need to begin to review the experiences with the objective of documenting some useful suggestions and making observations in regard to the process. A certain sadness began to prevail and members began to find it extremely difficult to come up with intimate suggestions and analyses. They began to solicit personal materials from each other and began to want to get to know about certain key members in the group. They especially wanted the leader to share much of his own past experiences, and would frequently ask him to make conclusions and interpretations about how the group had progressed and what it had accomplished. He spent a good portion of the remaining sessions gathering together and organizing material regarding the group into some coherent whole and then presenting it to the members for processing. He also brought many written process notes to share with the various members, and would ask members to respond in a personal way to many of his observations. Members were repeatedly reluctant, however, to analyze, but continued to offer many personal observations and expressions of their feelings. They seemed uninterested in intellectually expressing an understanding of what they had learned or what they had found lacking in the group. As the final moments approached, members began to express an appreciation for the experience that they had had. They also reported a great deal of previously undiscussed socializing that had taken place outside the group. In the last session they gathered around the leader and very affectionately departed, asking him if he would someday write a book about the materials and the experiences that had evolved.

Discussion

The group moved in stages. The beginning was characterized by considerable enthusiasm and activity — a universal feeling of pleasure in being a member and a strong wish to get things going. Everyone seemed to believe that the group would be a great success, and they felt a certain specialness in participating in such a unique venture. As the initial structure began to appear less useful and appealing, bewilderment, irritation, and disappointment set in. The members groped about for ways of relating to each other in the face of fears, suspicions, prejudices and stereotyped ideas. Some scattered as a means of defending themselves against the feelings and attitudes that the experience had provoked. Under the guidance of sensitive and strong leadership, a structure and climate was imposed on the group that brought the members back and encouraged free expression without fear of meeting anticipated rebuffs and punishment for openness of communication. A milieu of trust and warmth began to form and members were noted to accept differences in their fellow members less negatively. They ultimately experienced feelings of warmth, compassion, understanding, and admiration for one another and discovered innumerable areas of common concern that they did not think possible.

This experiment clearly parallels the experiences reported by a group of people of shared values and life styles upon entering a new reality at variance

with their own. Certain conflicts ensue and a restructing of reality is necessary
to bring oneself into some sort of equilibrium with the new situation. The conflict and the process of reconciliation give rise to a characteristic personality
organization and pattern of behavior which seems to develop in stages.

The parallel in adjustment patterns of this group with those of new immi-
grant groups which the author has studied is striking. These studies demonstrate
that a set of very specific stages characterize the accomodation or lack of adaptation to Boston for this migrant population. As it bears on understanding the
group, as well as Hispanic and other neighborhood immigrants, this material will
be briefly discussed here. The process was called the Sociocultural Disruption
Syndrome experience of the migrants and can be divided into four periods or
phases.

Initial Period

The *initial period* is the time of settling of the Spanish-speaking person in Boston.
It is characterized by: (1) feelings of euphoria and general well-being; (2) a certain
desire to get things moving; (3) confinement to the immediate vicinity and almost
exclusive attention to basic needs, such as food and shelter, and (4) a heightened
time perception of the immediate past, a certain introspection of a new, fresh self
and a continual self-justification of one's decision to migrate. It is at this time
that the Spanish-speaking are particularly receptive to outside influences, since
they are unfamiliar with the ways of the "Mainland" and impressed with and/or
proud of their adopted home. This is the time when steps could ideally be taken to
introduce the migrants to an unfamiliar setting, and facilitate their settlement. No
such activity, however, takes place for most Spanish-speaking migrants and this
failure leads to attendant psychological adjustments in the next stage.

Period of Awareness

In this *period of discovery,* the great disparities between the two cultures becomes
evident. These differences are often dramatically brought home to Spanish-speaking
migrants as they note the value systems, customs, and guideposts for interpersonal
relationships of the people they encounter in this new setting. Traditional roles, such
as between male and female, and the family and its structure are reexamined, often
leading to conflicts and confusion.

The new migrants become painfully aware of loss; whether physical — in the
form of property, jobs, and so forth, left behind; or human — beloved relatives
and friends who remained back home; or inability to function as they once did
because their ideas, skills, know-how, and ways of survival often have little relevance or utility in a highly educated and industrialized society. In short, mi-

grants have their rude awakening as they realize that life in the United States is
no bed of roses, especially for poor, rural-oriented, uneducated minorities, and
that Americans are just not that receptive to their being here in the first place.

Period of Devitalization

Out of this period comes the *period of devitalization* characterized by general
feelings of helplessness which often express themselves symptomatically in
obsessive defenses in the form of exaggerated concern for self, others, or the
environment. These "symptoms" (not disease, necessarily) can have both negative and positive benefits, depending on whether they are used as crutches to
excuse one's inability to cope or as a means to spur one to achieve the fourth
stage.

Young Spanish-speaking persons often assert their militancy and pride in
their heritage, and return the hostility of white and even black Americans. Or
they may engage in vandalism, crime, and drug traffic as a result of their difficulties in coming to terms with their oppressive environment. Older people, concerned with themselves, can become withdrawn and hostile or present with com-
pulsive behavior; somatic complaints are common as a defense mechanism. These
complaints may be grouped in three areas: (1) generalized fatigue; (2) systemic
complaints confined to particular areas of the body such as headaches, respira-
tory ailments, or problems with the stomach; and (3) the "wandering organ
syndrome," wherein the systemic complaint cured one day is soon replaced by
a new ailment in another body system.

The preoccupation with others can lead to an excessive suspicion of others,
especially those who do not belong to the tightly defined "clan," and even
paranoia; those predisposed to these reactions will fabricate all sorts of bugaboos
in order to cover up their inability to cope with their environment. On the positive side, however, the preoccupation with others may lead a parent to spend
much more time with his or her children in order that the latter at least will be
able to successfully attain the revitalization stage described below.

The excessive concern for the environment is often seen in a preoccupation
with such physical entities as the city itself, the apartment one lives in, or the
particular neighborhood. Complaints are frequent — whether against crime in
the streets, the welfare system, community leaders and the agencies they represent, or the inefficiency of garbage disposal. The general feeling is that "things
would not be so bad if one were not so hampered by physical inefficiency, lassi-
tude, or oppression of the external environment."

Period of Revitalization

Finally, one comes to the *revitalization stage,* the final determinant of successful immigration, which results in psychological and emotional equipping of oneself to deal realistically with society. Failure to achieve this stage may be seen in return to the homeland by some, perhaps to try again; in alcoholism among men who cannot or will not try anymore; in women with obsessive and somatic complaints; or in serious psychiatric disorders which remove people as functional members of their community.

The findings of these studies were presented to the group described previously in great detail shortly after it reestablished itself, and efforts were being made to begin anew with some comprehensive statement of purpose. It is of interest that these findings were enthusiastically accepted and seen as personally significant. A warm and moving period of sharing personal histories followed which characterized the remaining sessions. The parallel adjustment patterns of the group and the immigrants they served was striking and presented a useful learning opportunity.

Conclusion

The project seemed to provide an excellent means of training practitioners in understanding and resolving intergroup conflict. It proved successful in recreating as closely as possible the emotions and stresses inherent in such phenomena as migration, culture conflict, and the effects of social class mobility on professional identity. The deliberate structuring of the group to reproduce the various personal interchanges and experiences one would encounter in neighborhood clinical work was particularly useful. The key to the success of the group seemed to rest on the authority and structure the group leader provided, and the fact that the experience was given as an accredited course. The participants were rewarded for their efforts not only with personal growth, but with legitimate University credits that were meaningful and symbolic both inside and outside their immediate working environment.

The group responded because it gained from the experience an intellectual and emotional insight into the various sides that characterize all intergroup conflict. It allowed the participants to share an adventure that was intense, real, and vital to each of them. They all were personally witnessing the unfolding drama of the massive migrations of the Spanish-speaking to the large urban areas of the East coast. For a brief period of time, the group captured a rich and complex piece of living history; it studied it in a unique way and learned a great deal.

References

Brody, E.B., Ed. *Behavior in New Environments: Adaptation of Migrant Populations*. Beverly Hills, California: Sage Publications, 1970.

Durkin, H.E. The Group Therapy Movement, *Psych. Annals*, Vol. III, #3, March, 1972, p. 14.

Erikson, E.H., Identity and Uprootedness in Our Time, *Insight and Responsibility*, New York: W.W. Norton, 1964, pp 81-109.

Fitzpatrick, J.P., *Puerto Rican Americans: The Meaning of Migration to the Mainland*, Englewood Cliffs, N.J.; Prentice-Hall, 1971.

Jansen, C.J., Ed. *Readings in the Sociology of Migration*, New York: Pergamon Press, 1970.

Jiminez, R.L., *The Sociocultural Disruptive Syndrome of the Spanish-Speaking Migrant: Mental Health Issues in the Spanish-speaking Series*. South End Community Health Center, Boston, 1973. (Unpublished monograph used as text in course Titled: Culture Conflict and Mental Health. Boston University 1973-1975.)

Padilla, A.M. and Aranda, P. *Latino Mental Health: Bibliography and Abstracts*, DHEW pub. # (HSM) 73-9144 U.S. Govt. Printing Office, 1974.

— *Latino Mental Health: A Review of the Literature*. DHEW Pub. # (HSM) 73-9143 U.S. Govt. Printing Office, 1973.

Rosenbaum, M. and Berger, M. *Group Psychotherapy and Group Function*. New York: Basic Books, 1963.

Seward G. *Psychotherapy and Culture Conflict*. New York: The Ronald Press, 1956.

Social Aspects of Alienation: An Annotated Bibliography PHS Pub. #1978 U.S. Govt. Printing Office, April, 1969.

Sorokin, P.A., *Society, Culture and Personality: Their Structure and Dynamics*. New York: Harper and Bro., 1947.

Training Methodology, Part I: Background and Research: An Annotated Bibliography on Inservice Training for Key Professionals and for Allied Professionals in Community Mental Health. DHEW Pub. #1862, Part I, U.S. Govt. Printing Office, 1968.

Tyhurst, L. Displacement and Migration: A Study in Social Psychiatry. *American J. of Psych.*, Feb. 1951.

Weinberg, A.A., *Migration and Belonging*. The Hague: Martinus Nijhoff, 1961.

Wolberg, L.R., Experimental Groups. Can They Enhance Adaptation?, *Psych. Annals*, Vol. II, #3, March, 1972.

Epilogue

17 Facing the Nation: Some Issues and Answers for Neighborhood Psychiatry

Lee B. Macht and *Donald J. Scherl*

This is a time of transition in the practice of mental health. Of such periods, Nikos Kazantzakis, writing on another subject, makes reference to an ancient Chinese statement: "I curse you; may you live in an important age". [1] In psychiatry, this burden falls to us much as it did to the psychoanalytic practitioners of the mid-1900s and to the early founders of moral treatment in the mid-1800s.

With respect first to the more recent group, the mid-1900s saw the flowering and expansion of concepts of intrapsychic process and etiology in mental illness. That era and those formative ideas have shaped generations of Americans, indeed, of people throughout the world. It has affected the ways in which we look at our children; the ways in which we not only relate to one another but also the ways in which we conceive of our relationships; the ways in which we understand the motivations of others as well as the terms and formulas that guide our thinking and knowing of others — in our own society and across national boundaries. The core psychoanalytic concepts have had a pervasive impact; like the unconscious, they are easy to lose sight of.

The founders of the moral treatment movement in the first half of nineteenth century America were also pioneers in altering both the way in which the mentally ill were treated and the way in which they were thought about. Theirs was the high point in the development of humane, hospital-based care for the mentally ill. In some ways our present circumstances bear a greater similarity to this earlier era. Like theirs, ours may represent a watershed in the evolution of a new context for treatment — that of community-based care. A good deal can be learned from this earlier experience that bears on the question of whether or not our current progress will endure. Like moral psychiatry, neighborhood psychiatric practice is humanistic in orientation and focused upon individual value in a social context.

The moral treatment movement in psychiatry ebbed as a result of a series of developments [2,3,4] including: the inability of the hospital system to care for the wave of nineteenth century immigrants; an evolving sense of pessimism with regard to the successful treatment of mental illness in comparison to other medical illnesses which increasingly were the beneficiaries of the new "scientific medicine"; the death of the early group of enlightened leaders who failed to leave behind trained and educated successors; an economic recession; and the shift of responsibility to the already overburdened and understaffed mental health system of that time (hospitals) from the correctional system (jails) and the welfare system (poor houses).

Neighborhood psychiatry faces different though not dissimilar forces which give pause to those who hope this new form of humanistic psychiatric practice will endure. There is, for example, still but a small cadre of practitioners, highlighting a crucial need for training and education in this field. There is a need for practitioners to describe their programs and their work, much as did the hospital superintendents who gave birth to moral treatment in psychiatry. The danger exists that as neighborhood psychiatry continues to grow and to improve its linkages with general medicine for fiscal and programmatic reasons, like moral treatment, it may lose its individualistic and humanistic underpinnings, neglecting in the process the study and treatment of the whole person in a family and neighborhood context. There is a clear need for neighborhood psychiatry to continue to maintain its humanism in the broadest sense. Finally, there is the need for assessment and evaluation if these services, which seem so beneficial on face evidence, are to demonstrate their efficacy in ways which the scientific and governmental communities will accept and understand.

We have defined the field of neighborhood psychiatry as one in which the range of clinical and community mental health functions are practiced within discrete, natural sociopolitical and geographical areas or neighborhoods. This field of special practice is related to other forms of mental health service delivery, but distinctly different in its focus on the neighborhood and its formal and informal networks, on collaborative service delivery, on an attempt to integrate clinical with population-centered approaches to mental health services, and on the linkages that create an organized system of care rather than a series of episodic interventions. Whether neighborhood psychiatry in the last quarter of the twentieth century will constitute a continuing new field or whether it represents simply a movement remains an open question. Whether the provision of mental health services in neighborhood settings is merely a passing phenomenon in the long history of man's attempts to assist his neighbors in need, or whether it represents a lasting contribution will only be answered in the future; the current era is too close to assess this accurately. Yet we believe that a trend is discernible in support of the relative permanence of neighborhood psychiatric practice.

The trend toward neighborhood-based care was fostered by the proliferation of social service legislation which marked the 1960s. In 1963, for example, President Kennedy submitted the Community Mental Health Services Act to the Congress. The programmatic result has been the development of a network of community-based mental health services supported by Federal Staffing and Construction Grants. In the mid-sixties, catchment area mental health centers began to decentralize services into neighborhood settings concomitant with the neighborhood-based health and mental health programs emanating from the Office of Economic Opportunity. Three distinct patterns of neighborhood mental health service emerged over this decade: solo neighborhood psychiatric practice; neighborhood mental health services as a part of comprehensive local health or mental health centers or systems; and mental health services forming a part of neighborhood human service centers or networks.

By 1971 this new pattern in the delivery of mental health services had become an important element in the total mental health caregiving system. A body of experience was growing across the country upon which those involved in neighborhood psychiatry could begin to draw, as programs attempted increasingly to decentralize. But the 1970s also saw federal funds for comprehensive health and mental health services diminish, and it became necessary for local programs to seek out new funding sources. This led to attempts in many states to reallocate resources from state-supported mental hospitals and mental health centers to private nonprofit neighborhood facilities. Many programs also attempted to qualify for third-party reimbursements. Despite these fiscal obstacles, the trend toward decentralization of community mental health center services continued, consistent with the theoretical framework which evolved during the 1960s. This frame-work placed a high value on the location of services close to where people lived and on the need to integrate services into the natural sociopolitical units within which people really spend their time — their local communities.

Recent federal legislation has continued to foster this trend. The "Community Mental Health Center Amendments of 1975" [5], for example, reiterated the view that "community mental health care is the most effective and humane form of care for a majority of mentally ill individuals." The amendments made clear the view of the Congress that community mental health centers have had a major impact on "fostering coordination and cooperation between the various agencies responsible for mental health care which in turn has resulted in a decrease in overlapping services and more efficient utilization of available resources." Of particular importance to neighborhood psychiatry are those provisions of the amendments which encourage decentralization and local integration of services, and which call for provision of services in the most relevant possible setting:

The provision of comprehensive mental health services through a center shall be coordinated with the provision of services by other health and social service agencies (including state mental health facilities) in or serving the center's catchment area to insure that persons receiving services through the center have access to all such health and social services as they may require. The center's services A) may be provided at the center or satellite centers through the staff of the center or through appropriate arrangements with health professionals and others in the center's catchment area. B) shall be available and accessible to the residents of the area promptly, as appropriate, and in a manner which preserves human dignity and assures continuity and high-quality care and which overcomes geographical, cultural, linguistic and economic barriers to the receipt of services, [5].

These amendments, together with certain provisions of the Federal "Health Planning and Resources Development Act of 1972" (P.L. 93-641), provide a public policy context for the further growth and evolution of neighborhood psychiatry. Looking to the future, current planning for national health insurance appears to include provisions that would allow (indeed encourage) reimbursement of mental health services within neighborhood settings.

At the state level we find it striking that the commonwealth of Massachusetts, for example, in its new "Five-Year Plan for Mental Health Services" [6] (written as a requirement of PL94-63, the newest federal community mental health act) fully endorses and embodies the neighborhood approach throughout; for example: in discussing the NIMH categorical services the Massachusetts Plan states:

One important example of how the "twelve essential services" model does not fit Department of Mental Health plans and expectations is the integrated Human Service approach at the neighborhood level. *In this plan the Department of Mental Health is assuming leadership in providing mental health and retardation services which are integrally linked to human services networks organized at neighborhood levels* (their emphasis). Although this approach has already been successfully implemented in some catchment areas to some degree, the Department's goal is to elaborate and extend this approach significantly in the next five years. This shift away from an emphasis on narrowly defined mental health and retardation services at the area (catchment area) level to the integrated human services model at the neighborhood level, grows out of the Department's deepening understanding of the problems and needs of its clients.

This broad statement of public policy goes further to state:

Many activities of mental health and retardation services must be directed and take place at the neighborhood level (their emphasis) not only do clients live in neighborhoods; many community support networks and institutions (the school, the neighborhood health center, the church) operate at this level. The presence of mental health services within neighborhoods, particularly if these are imbedded in more general helping contexts (e.g. a neighborhood human services or health center) and provided by both paid workers and volunteers from the community as well as helping professionals, greatly reduces many barriers to integration such as geographic and social distance and clients' fears of stigmatization. These factors also promote prevention, early detection and outreach, facilitating relations with neighborhood natural support systems and encouraging citizens and professionals to become involved with community issues and concerns. Although some catchment areas may correspond to such neighborhoods or "natural" communities, most catchment areas are more extensive. *In such cases, Area Directors and Area Boards must address the smaller neighborhoods in their plans and service delivery systems.* (their emphasis).

There are strong, enlightened and progressive, statements of public mental health policy which other states can emulate.

These recent developments involving federal and state health and public policy initiatives, planning, and resource allocations, along with the continuing commitment on the part of citizens and the professions, lead us to be optimistic concerning the future of neighborhood psychiatry as an important component in the delivery of mental health services in America. While we believe this for some of the reasons just cited, we also believe that its future is uncertain.

It may be well to consider some of the issues which neighborhood psychiatry will have to face over the next years. Perhaps the greatest challenge to this approach lies outside the usually cited issues of service delivery, service financing, and manpower availability. Instead it resides in the lack of commitment of communities and neighborhoods to personal involvement in mental health problems — involvement of people in a community or neighborhood, one with another. We do not lack conceptualizations of neighborhood psychiatric practice; rather, we face a breakdown of the neighborhood as a social unit. A good deal has been written about the break-down of the family unit. But on a larger canvas, neighborhoods and communities have been undergoing similar deteriorative change. Lack of interest of persons within communities and lack of a sense of responsibility for one another mean that the disabled, the chronically impaired, and of course the mentally ill and the retarded are extruded. Instead of being considered as impaired members of a social grouping who require special attention, these persons are placed in the category of outgroup or nongroup members. Where this is so, it becomes impossible to establish group residences or halfway houses, to find foster parents for children in need, or to establish a sense of community responsibility for the healthy growth and development of the neighborhood's children. Where the community feels no sense of responsibility toward its own members, the sick and the well, neighborhood psychiatry cannot flourish, indeed can scarcely subsist. Neighborhood mental health workers cannot substitute for, cannot create, and cannot exist without a caring neighborhood.

This lack is part of a larger issue. Just as the success of neighborhood psychiatric practice depends upon an existing (or at least available) sense of neighborhood or community, it also depends in large measure on the resolution in society of broader underlying issues. Matters of "the quality of life" bear critically upon local mental health practice, particularly primary prevention and the care of the chronically disabled. We refer here to matters such as income maintenance, adequate nutrition in order to avoid developmental attrition in children, adequate housing, safe neighborhoods, and so forth. We do not view the mental health professions as solely responsible for the resolution of these issues. Instead, we point to them as matters which underlie, in a fundamental sense, the ability of individuals and families to cope with the intrapsychic and social stresses to which they are subject. In our view, the practitioner should not expect local preventive interventions, however creative, to have any major impact until these other issues are faced. The fact that these matters remain unresolved does not remove from the neighborhood psychiatric practitioner the obligation of dealing with episodic and clinical mental illness as it occurs. Those in the field of neighborhood mental health practice should be able to clearly differentiate social prevention as an ideal from daily remedial work as a practical necessity. We also recognize that while resolution of these underlying social problems is a necessity if preventive interventions are to be successful, the other major avenue of prevention now receiving increasing recognition involves the willingness of individuals to reduce their own risk-taking behavior. In areas such as drinking, drug use, nutrition, exercise, and others, people need to learn how to protect their health and mental health. Unless people assume this sort of responsibility for themselves, there is relatively little of a preventive nature that can be accomplished. Our role is to help people become willing to follow reasonable health and mental health practices.

One core element in establishing neighborhood-based services for communities in which there is some sense of interpersonal responsibility involves the formation of adequate human support systems and the linkage of these systems into the pattern of neighborhood psychiatric practice. It is at the neighborhood level of social organization that many natural support systems already exist or can be developed. Understanding how service systems can be integrated and also how human support systems can be developed merits further study. While these aspects of the field have evolved considerably, important issues of accountability, planning, confidentiality, continuity of care, "turf" and power, and values and attitudes require additional attention. Equally important, considerably more must be learned about how to make neighborhood centers integral parts of the communities they serve without interferring with necessary linkages to formal backup resources, on the one hand, and to informal neighborhood caregiving networks, on the other. Human support systems and linked networks of services are of particular importance to those who are chronically impaired. They form the bedrock of the process of "deinstitutionalization" if the movement of patients from institutions to community is to take place with any success. Neighborhood psychiatry stands in the greatest jeopardy if it does not provide care for the "sickest" and most handicapped residents of a neighborhood — and if the neighborhood will not allow it to provide that care.

The development of support systems of the type described would appear to depend increasingly upon the ways in which public funds and private services are linked. Mental health services are supported in very substantial part by public monies. This includes both the publicly operated state hospital service system which has evolved over the past hundred years and the community mental health centers and mental health clinics which have developed especially since World War II. While the private sector includes many voluntary (nonprofit) facilities and services, it also includes private practitioners and proprietary mental hospitals. The melding of these various service elements into a care system which is neighborhood-responsive yet publicly financed (especially as the reality of national health insurance approaches) presents a major challenge for the next decade or more. It is especially important, in our view, that neighborhood services form strong and integrated linkages with other elements of the primary health care system.

The list of issues which our field will face over the next years seems in some ways endless. We have chosen to highlight matters of primary mental health care service and public education, the allied issue of prevention, the survival of this new subspecialty field of psychiatry, the development of human support systems and of linked service systems, and the importance of neighborhood and community. Implicit in our discussion has been a concern with prevention on the one side and assistance for the chronically disabled on the other. We are concerned in particular that evolving primary care systems not lose sight of the deinstitutionalized mentally ill patient, the mentally retarded individual, and the need to focus particular attention on the healthy growth and development of children. While each of these matters merits additional specific attention, we choose to end with a definitional question. It involves the issue of which patients and which problems will respond best to a neighborhood psychiatry model and which are better left to clinics, hospitals, and mental health centers. This type of careful clinical evaluative research is basic to the development of a rational service system with rationally allocated resources. It needs to be undertaken now.

As scientists we recognize the absence of definitive evaluative research in most areas of psychiatric practice, of which neighborhood psychiatry is no exception. Our confidence in the future of this field of practice is as much personal, therefore, as it is professional. Each of us has participated in delivering neighborhood mental health services and each of us has seen them work. While our scientific bent inclines us to urge caution in awaiting the results of careful research studies, our own experience leads us to think that clinical choices favoring neighborhood practice can be made now. Definitive studies will be a long time in coming. We share with our colleagues a sense of having turned a corner in establishing a model of mental health service of some lasting value.

References

1. Bennis, W.G. A Funny Thing Happened on the Way to the Future, In *Psychology and the Problems of Society,* Korten, F., Cook, S. Lacey, J. (Eds.) American Psychological, Inc. Washington, D.C. 1970 pp. 431-450.
2. Bockoven, J.S., *Moral Treatment in American Psychiatry.* New York; Springer Publishing Co. 1963.
3. Caplan, R.B. *Psychiatry and the Community in Nineteenth Century America.* New York: Basic Books, Inc. 1969.
4. Macht, L.B. Community Psychiatry. In Textbook of Psychiatry to be published by Harvard University Press, Edited by Armand Nicholi.
5. Community Mental Health Amendments of 1975. PL 94-348, Title III.

6. Massachusetts Department of Mental Health five year plan for mental health services. Commonwealth of Massachusetts. Department of Mental Health, September 24, 1976.

Index

About the Contributors

James C. Beck, M.D., Ph.D.   Assistant Professor of Psychiatry at The Cambridge Hospital, Harvard Medical School and Chief of Community Consultation and Research, Department of Psychiatry, The Cambridge Hospital.

William J. Bicknell, M.D., M.P.H.   Professional Associate, Family Health Care, Inc., Washington, D.C.; Senior Consultant in Long Term Care Program Development, Harvard School of Public Health; Formerly Commissioner of Public Health, Commonwealth of Massachusetts.

Jonathan F. Borus, M.D.   Assistant Professor of Psychiatry, Harvard Medical School; Director of Residency Training, Department of Psychiatry, Massachusetts General Hospital; Chief Psychiatric Consultant, North End Community Health Center, Boston; Director, Social and Community Psychiatry Subspecialty Training Program, Massachusetts General Hospital and Erich Lindemann Mental Health Center, Boston.

Jack R. Ewalt, M.D.   Director Mental Health and Behavioral Science, United States Veterans Administration Headquarters; Bullard Professor Emeritus, Harvard Medical School.

Sandra Sutherland Fox, Ph.D.   Chair, Undergraduate Program in Social Work, National Catholic School of Social Services, Catholic University of America, Washington, D.C.

Chester D. Haskell   Director of Public Management Training, National Center for Urban Ethnic Affairs.

Roberto L. Jiminez, M.D.   Psychiatrist-in-Chief, South End Community Health Center, Boston, MA; Assistant Professor of Psychiatry Boston University School of Medicine; Clinical Instructor in Psychiatry, Harvard Medical School; Massachusetts Mental Health Center; Lecturer Criminal Justice, Northeastern University College of Criminal Justice.

Gerald L. Klerman, M.D.   Professor of Psychiatry, Harvard Medical School; Director of Stanley Cobb Research Laboratories, Department of Psychiatry, Massachusetts General Hospital.

Richard D. Kluft, M.D.   Associate in Psychiatry, Institute of Pennsylvania Hospital.

Robert L. Leopold, M.D.   Professor of Psychiatry, School of Medicine; Professor of Health Care Systems, Wharton School — University of Pennsylvania; Consulting Psychiatrist, American Friends Service Committee, Inc.

Orlando B. Lightfoot, M.D.   Senior Psychiatrist, Solomon C. Fuller Mental Health Center; Associate Professor, Boston University School of Medicine; Associate Visiting Psysician, University Hospital; Senior Psychiatrist, Boston City Hospital; Staff Psychiatrist, South End Community Health Center; Director, Adult Ambulatory Services, Boston University School of Medicine.

Jancis V.F. Long, M.A.   Clinical Psychologist, The Cambridge Hospital; Teaching Fellow, Harvard University.

Eugene L. Lowenkopf, M.D.   Director, Residency Training, Kirby Psychiatric Center; Assistant Clinical Professor of Psychiatry, New York Medical College.

Richard G. Morrill, M.D.   Associate Professor, Department of Psychiatry and Department of Community Medicine at Boston University Medical School; Director of Mental and Social Health at Roxbury Comprehensive Community Health Center; Director of Department of Mental Health at Uphams Corner Health Center.

Arthur J. Naparstek, Ph.D.   Director, University of Southern California, Washington Public Affairs Center; Previously Director of Policy and Program Development, National Center for Urban Ethnic Affairs.

Martin M. Norman, Ph.D.   Program Director, Jamaica Plain Outreach Program; Senior Staff Psychologist at Judge Baker Guidance Center and Children's Hospital Medical Center; Staff Affiliation, Massachusetts Mental Health Center.

Diana Paul   Psychiatric Coordinator of the Martin L. King, Jr. Health Center.

Chester M. Pierce, M.D.   Professor of Education and Psychiatry in the Faculty of Medicine and at the Graduate School of Education, Harvard University, Cambridge, MA.

Lee C. Reich, Ph.D.   Clinical Psychologist, Laboure Center, South Boston; Assistant Clinical Professor of Psychiatry, Tufts University School of Medicine.

Julius B. Richmond, M.D.   Professor of Child Psychiatry and Human Development and Professor of Preventive and Social Medicine at Harvard Medical School; Director of the Judge Baker Guidance Center; Psychiatrist-In-Chief at the Children's Hospital Medical Center.

James E. Sabin, M.D.   Staff of the Harvard Community Health Plan; Clinical Instructor in Psychiatry, Harvard Medical School.

Diana Chapman Walsh   Senior Program Associate, Massachusetts Department of Public Health; Assistant Project Coordinator, Office of Extramural Health Programs, Harvard School of Public Health.

About the Editors

Lee B. Macht is Director of Clinical Services, The Cambridge Hospital, Department of Psychiatry and Director of Clinical Services, The Cambridge-Somerville Mental Health and Retardation Center and Associate Professor of Psychiatry, Harvard Medical School. He received the A.B. from Princeton University in 1957 and the M.D. from Harvard Medical School in 1961. Dr. Macht obtained adult and child psychiatric training at Massachusetts Mental Health Center and has served as Principal Psychiatrist and Deputy Medical Director of the Job Corps and as a senior psychiatrist and consultant to the Office of Economic Opportunity. Dr. Macht has also served as Commissioner of Mental Health in Massachusetts and has performed research and written on several areas of clinical and community psychiatry.

Donald J. Scherl is Associate Professor of Psychiatry at Harvard Medical School. He received his medical degree from Harvard University and his bachelor's degree, summa cum laude, from Yale University. He is Director of Outpatient and Liaison Psychiatry and Associate Chief of the Department of Psychiatry, Children's Hospital Medical Center and Associate Director of the Judge Baker Guidance Center, Boston, Massachusetts. From 1971 to 1975, Dr. Scherl served as Undersecretary of Human Services for the Commonwealth of Massachusetts after having spent four years as Director of Community Mental Health Services, Massachusetts Mental Health Center, Harvard Medical School.

Steven Sharfstein is Acting Director of the Mental Health Services Division of the National Institute of Mental Health. He received the A.B. from Dartmouth College in 1964 and the M.D. from the Albert Einstein College of Medicine in 1968. Dr. Sharfstein received a Masters in Public Administration from the John F. Kennedy School of Government at Harvard University in 1973. He obtained psychiatric training at the Massachusetts Mental Health Center and has served as Director of Mental Health Services at the Brookside Park Family Life Center. Dr. Sharfstein has recently served as the Director of Program analysis and Evaluation in the Office of Program Development and Analysis of the NIMH and has had a Mental Health Career Development Fellowship.